OXFORD MEDICAL PUBLICATIONS

THE CANCER PREVENTION MANUAL

Simple rules to reduce the risks

By the same author

Cancer Explained, Wakefield Press, Adelaide, South Australia, 1997, and Gill and Macmillan, Dublin, by arrangement.

All About Prostate Cancer, Oxford University Press, Melbourne, 2000.

All About Breast Cancer, Oxford University Press, Melbourne, 2001.

THE CANCER PREVENTION MANUAL

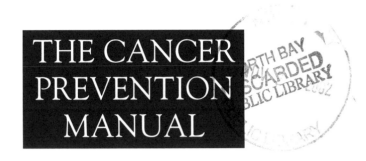

Simple rules to reduce the risks

Professor Fred Stephens

AM, MD, MS, FRCS (Ed), FACS, FRACS

Emeritus Professor and former Head of
Department of Surgery, University of Sydney

Consultant Emeritus in Surgical Oncology
Sydney Hospital and The Royal Prince Alfred
Hospital, Sydney, Australia

Former Senior Registrar in Surgery, University of
Aberdeen Teaching Hospitals, Scotland

Former Visiting Fulbright Professor, University of
California, San Francisco

Former President, The International Society For
Regional Cancer Therapy

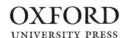

OXFORD
UNIVERSITY PRESS

OXFORD

UNIVERSITY PRESS

Great Clarendon Street, Oxford OX2 6DP

Oxford University Press is a department of the University of Oxford.
It furthers the University's objective of excellence in research, scholarship,
and education by publishing worldwide in

Oxford   New York

Auckland   Bangkok   Buenos Aires   Cape Town   Chennai
Dar es Salaam   Delhi   Hong Kong   Istanbul   Karachi   Kolkata
Kuala Lumpur   Madrid   Melbourne   Mexico City   Mumbai   Nairobi
São Paulo   Shanghai   Taipei   Tokyo   Toronto

and an associated company in Berlin

Oxford is a registered trade mark of Oxford University Press
in the UK and in certain other countries

Published in the United States
by Oxford University Press Inc., New York

© Oxford University Press, 2002

British Library Cataloguing in Publication Data
(Data available)

Library of Congress Cataloging in Publication Data

(Data available)

ISBN 0 19 852532 X

10 9 8 7 6 5 4 3 2 1

Typeset by Cepha Imaging Pvt Ltd, India

Printed in Great Britain
on acid-free paper by Biddles Ltd, Guildford & King's Lynn

Contents

Contents

Acknowledgements

I am delighted to acknowledge that much of the incentive and stimulus for writing this book came from my daughter Jenny. As a mother Jenny wanted information about cancer prevention to be readily available in a book, both as a guide in the care of her own family and as a guide for all mothers in care of their families.

My wife, Sheilagh, my daughter Katriona, and my son Peter were especially helpful in reading the manuscript and ensuring that the language and explanations were clear and easily understood by people who do not necessarily have a medical background.

My friends in the Audio-visual department of The Royal Prince Alfred Hospital, Sydney, are always helpful in preparing illustrations. Mr Bob Haynes has special skills in converting my rough diagrams into meaningful illustrations.

I acknowledge with gratitude Dr John Knight's encouragement of my interest in writing books to meet the needs of people from different backgrounds in coming to terms with worries about cancer. In private life Dr Knight is a highly experienced general practitioner in a Sydney suburb but in public life, using the *nom de plume* 'Dr James Wright', he is a prominent medical broadcaster and medical columnist.

Dedication

I am glad to dedicate this book to my family. As a husband, father, father-in-law and grandfather it is a constant delight to have such a devoted family, every member of which I am very proud and love dearly. I am also privileged to have a large, close and warm extended family of brothers, sisters, in-laws, nieces, nephews and cousins. They have always been encouraging and supportive of my work.

One of life's real blessings is to be a member of such a close, warm and caring family group all of whom have followed a wonderful example set by my parents, Dorys and Hedley Stephens of the little village of Kurmond, New South Wales. My parents were poor in physical possessions but rich in their love.

I am pleased to honour my late and much loved brother, Bruce, who encouraged me to write this book especially to help people with young families like his own.

Preface

There are probably few occupations where the objective is to make one's job redundant, but this is clearly the aim of all cancer research workers.

In over 30 years of clinical and research work in cancer I have derived a great deal of satisfaction from being able to treat people troubled by cancers, and from investigating and improving methods of cancer care and treatment. I have made many friends with similar interests in the health professions the world over and amongst patients who have entrusted themselves to my care. Fortunately most of those patients have done well; for those with incurable disease it has usually been possible to extend their expected lifespan and to help make the time remaining to them more comfortable. Their trust and friendship has been reward in itself.

However, like all researchers in this field, my greatest ambition is to make my work unnecessary.

The best thing to do about cancer is to do everything possible to prevent the disease. This is the preferred objective of all cancer research workers, but it has to be a three-way process:

1. First, the medical profession and other scientists and health professionals must find ways and means through lifestyles and other practices, whatever they may be, to eliminate or reduce the risk of cancer.

2. Second it is up to those at risk, and that is all of us, to help and encourage changes in our lifestyles

or otherwise put desirable community changes into practice. Clearly an additional responsibility for such changes rests with lawmakers and others in authority.

3. The third essential ingredient is to achieve effective communication between those in the above two groups. This will ensure that those in a position to put the changes into practice (administrators and each of us as individuals) are given all of the most important available information and thus are well informed as to what can and should be done.

The objective of this book is to help fill this third role; that is, to inform people and authorities in clear, honest and, where necessary, forceful terms, of changes that can be effected to reduce the risk of cancer.

The structure of this book

This book is written in five sections, each of which may be read separately according to the special interest of the reader.

Section 1 is an introduction explaining what cancers are and what causes them. It also explains some of the science and philosophy of cancer prevention and roles that can be played by those of us who try to do something about it.

The information in sections 2, 3 and 4 overlaps somewhat. Section 2 is a general introduction to the problem of cancer, the different kinds of cancer and how cancers can be classified into different types.

Section 3 identifies important aspects of lifestyle practices that people can change or modify to reduce their risk of cancers in general. It contains specific help on self-examination, cancer screening tests and medical advice, and discusses the types of cancer that can presently be influenced by attention to these practices. Conditions that might predispose to malignancy are also outlined. Finally, areas where government legislation protects citizens, particularly in industrial practices, are discussed.

Section 4 deals with specific cancers. Most of the cancers described here will have been mentioned in section 3, but for those readers interested in one particular type of cancer, information about prevention of the most common cancers will be summarized in this section. These are the cancers with a risk that can be reduced, to a greater or lesser degree, by modification or change in lifestyle or other practices.

Section 5 summarizes the nature of cancer, lifestyle changes that can reduce the risk of certain cancers, and future directions of research for cancer prevention and treatment.

Section 1

Introduction

What is cancer?

A cancer is a continuous, unwanted, uncontrolled and destructive growth of abnormal cells that have developed from the body's own previously normal cells. When tissues grow in infants and young people, when injured or worn out cells are replaced, when hair grows, new blood cells are needed or lining cells of skin or the food passages are lost, they are replaced by nearby or underlying cells dividing to make new cells. When growing has been completed, healing has taken place, or worn out cells have been replaced, an inbuilt braking system normally stops cell division until new cells are needed once again.

A cancer begins when something has changed in one or more of the cells in the body, causing them to continue to divide and form new cells that are not wanted. Like a car with no brakes, the cells are out of control. The new, unwanted cells grow and penetrate into other tissues, damaging them. Whatever it is that normally stops the cells from growing when no more are needed has failed.

Cancer cells may get into the bloodstream or into other vessels (lymphatic vessels) and travel to distant organs or tissues where they may get stuck and grow. The new growing cancer lumps are called secondary cancers or metastases. It is rather like the wind spreading the seeds of a weed in a garden; the weeds start to grow in other places. Just as weeds are more likely to grow in some soils than others, so cancer cells tend to grow more in some tissues. Throughout this process the body has lost control of the dividing cancerous cells.

The word *cancer* is Latin for 'crab', and at one time cancer was likened to a crab with claws that grew into the surrounding tissues, causing them damage. Despite many advances in its detection and treatment, after cardiovascular disease, cancer is the greatest killer of adults in Western countries.

The old axiom that prevention is better than cure is particularly relevant to cancer. With better knowledge of those factors associated with increased risk of cancer, cancer prevention is now a realistic approach. Most of the changes needed are in lifestyle, habits, and possibly living conditions. Success will depend very much upon their acceptance by each individual and by the community in general.

The medical profession and other health professionals can help inform and educate individuals and responsible organizations about measures that can be taken to help reduce the risks of cancer developing. Although in some areas important preventive measures are well known, for example avoiding tobacco smoking, there will always be resistance and denial from those with entrenched interests. With regard to some aspects of diet there is still room for discussion, speculation, debate, and further study, but we already possess some vital clues that merit attention and possible action. In other areas, little or nothing is known about what is causing the uncontrolled cell growth, and a great deal of further investigation is needed.

There is no doubt about the dangers of tobacco products and of smoking in general, nor about the risks of asbestos, of the practice of chewing betel nut, or of certain chemical agents such as phosphorus and the aniline dyes.

There is no doubt about the dangers of over exposure to ultraviolet light, X-rays, gamma rays and cosmic irradiation.

There is no doubt about the risks of certain pre-malignant conditions if left untreated, and of some viruses and other infestations.

It is becoming increasingly apparent that more attention should be given to diet and dietary ingredients. People who adhere to different dietary practices have different risks of some cancers. Although a good deal is known about these relationships, much has yet to be learnt about the most advantageous ingredients and how they might influence or depress tumour cell development or growth.

On the other hand this is no time for complacency. There is still a lot to be learnt and for many cancers prevention is still a dream. For any cancer, precise basic knowledge of the exact initiating process is still a mystery. We know that changes in genes are responsible for the continuing cancer cell growth, but much remains to be discovered about how and why these genetic changes take place, and how they might be modified or prevented. Exciting research in genetics and molecular biology offers the hope of unravelling some of these mysteries, but who knows where answers will come from tomorrow?

Meanwhile increased knowledge and understanding provide great opportunities for improvements in cancer prevention. So does earlier detection, together with more effective treatments. The opportunities are there and success will be assured if patients, researchers, practitioners, health organizations, and administrators work together. The greater the application, dedication, and cooperation, the greater will be the success. There is light at the end of this very dark tunnel.

This book is one writer's attempt to shine some of that light.

Section 2

An outline of the causes of cancer

About one in four or five Europeans, North Americans, Australians or New Zealanders will die of cancer, and the risk is similar in most other countries that keep records. Although diagnostic and treatment methods have improved and are constantly under study the overall death rates have remained pretty much the same; partly because people are living longer and most cancers become more common in older age groups.

Other than earlier detection and improved treatment methods, the greatest impact on the cancer problem lies in its prevention. For many cancers little is known about causes, but for some, causes or associations are well known and the risk of getting a particular type of cancer can be greatly reduced.

In general the causes of cancer fall into two broad groups—*congenital* and *acquired*. Until recently there has been little we can do about most of our inherited or congenital abnormalities, but the acquired problems are often either preventable or controllable.

Congenital and inherited causes

Congenital causes are generally regarded as those defects or abnormalities present at birth. Defects that develop later in life due to defects in genes inherited from parents are now included in this group, although they are more correctly referred to as *familial* or *genetic*. Genes that carry an increased cancer risk may be a feature of particular families or of particular races. Genes are present in all living cells. They are inherited from parents and are the basic tissue-building organizers of plant and animal life. Until recently it was assumed that we had to accept our genes as an unchangeable accident of life inherited from our parents. Little could be done about it, although sometimes precautions could be taken to prevent any inherited premalignant condition from developing into a cancer, usually by removing the premalignant tissue concerned before any malignant change had taken place. One example of this is an inherited genetic bowel condition called '*familial polyposis coli*'. A parent who has this condition will pass this gene on to 50 per cent of his or her children. Any child who inherits the gene will, later in life, develop polyps, that is, little lumps in the inside lining of the large bowel. Sooner or later at least one of these lumps will become a cancer. This almost always happens before the age of 40, but it can be prevented by an operation in which the whole large bowel is removed in all affected offspring before a cancer has developed.

The new science of genetic engineering allows a new approach in cancer prevention and treatment. In some cases, abnormal genes can be altered or replaced to reduce the risk of malignant cells developing.

The other much larger group of causes of cancer is known as the *acquired* group. Acquired causes of disease are those things—conditions or aspects of living or environment—that can result from something happening later in life. Some acquired causes of cancer such as smoking, excessive sunlight on white skin, particular types of diet or certain chemicals, are known or suspected, but others are as yet unknown. These are the conditions or causes or agents that people can do most about—either by ourselves, with the help of our doctors, or through responsible authorities like governments or councils. We need to learn to avoid these known or strongly suspected causes of cancer, in order to reduce the risk of getting a cancer. In Section 3 these lifestyle factors are examined as 'The seven S's of cancer prevention'.

Acquired causes of cancer

Inflammations

Some long-standing inflammations, especially of the large bowel (colon and rectum), may lead to cancer. Long-standing unhealed ulcers, stomach ulcers or simple skin ulcers, for example varicose ulcers that occur commonly on the lower legs, can sometimes develop malignant change. That is, changes can occur in their cells that can lead to cancer if the ulcers are left unhealed for some years. Other long-standing irritated or inflamed tissue from a variety of causes can also develop malignant change, as described below. In some cases (e.g. the large bowel) the specific cause of a long-standing or chronic inflammation may not yet be fully understood.

Micro-organisms—viruses, bacteria, fungus, parasites

Viruses

In animals some cancers are clearly linked to virus infection, but viruses are rarely direct causes of cancers in humans. Sometimes a virus can cause changes that can lead to cancer, e.g. the human *papilloma virus* or the AIDS virus. The human papilloma virus can cause papillomas of skin (see Figure 7, page 71) in either sex, and in women it can cause small papillomas or other changes in or near the cervix of the uterus (the entrance of the womb), or the vagina. In either case these papillomas can become malignant; that is, cancerous. The human papilloma virus can be transmitted by sexual intercourse and is now increasingly recognized as a factor in many cases of cancer of the cervix of the uterus. Attempts have been made to find an effective vaccine to protect against the human papilloma virus, especially for women at special risk. Some success has been reported, and it is expected that effective immunization will soon become available.

The AIDS virus weakens the natural protective defences of the body, and so can indirectly lead to cancer. Lymphoma (often described as a cancer of the immune system) will sometimes develop in AIDS patients. Kaposi's sarcoma, a cancer of soft tissues, is especially associated with the AIDS virus. Soft tissues are those tissues between skin and underlying bones—muscle, fat, blood vessels and nerves. Epstein–Barr virus is often associated with increased risk of cancer behind the nose, and is particularly prevalent in Hong Kong and some parts of China. A similar virus in tropical Africa and New Guinea has been linked to a cancer in children called Burkitt's lymphoma. The Epstein–Barr virus is spread by mosquitoes, so that people living in places where the virus is common could reduce their cancer risk by taking protective measures against mosquitoes.

Significant cancer-related viruses in South-East Asia—the hepatitis viruses, especially hepatitis B and hepatitis C—are now becoming more common in Europe, North America, Australia and New Zealand. Whilst they do not directly cause cancer, the inflammation they cause in the liver can develop into a liver cancer. These viruses can be spread by direct human contact, especially sexual contact, and also in contaminated food. For anyone at special risk, and this is now possibly everyone living in Australia, New Zealand, North America and Europe but certainly everyone travelling to Asia, protection by immunization against the hepatitis B virus is effective and is strongly recommended. Reliable protection against hepatitis C is not available at the time of writing, but several research groups are working on this need.

There has recently been some concern that the SV40 virus—usually associated with monkeys—may have contaminated early preparations of the anti-poliomyelitis Salk vaccine and thus may have been transmitted to people who were immunized in the 1960s. A small number of these people have since developed a range of unusual cancers, some of which contained SV40. It is still not known if there was any direct association between the virus and the cancers, but legislation has imposed strict precautions to avoid any possibility of this, or any similar contamination, taking place in preparation of vaccines or any other medications in the future.

Bacteria

Bacteria are rarely, if ever, directly responsible for causing cancer. They sometimes cause wounds or ulcers to fail to heal, and this chronic or long-standing inflamed tissue can sometimes develop malignant change, but this is not a direct effect of the bacteria. The *Helicobacter pylori* organism, a cause of gastric ulcers, has also been implicated in stomach cancer. It remains uncertain whether it is a direct cause of cancer or causes persistent inflammation or ulceration in which cancer can develop.

Fungus

Fungus infection, common in the mouth and throat or vagina in some people, does not directly cause cancer, but long term irritation and infection by a fungus can lead to abnormal white patches called *leukoplakia* (leukoplakia is Latin for white patches). Occasionally a cancer will develop in one or more of these white patches in the mouth or in the vagina.

Parasites

Like bacteria or fungus, parasites do not directly cause cancer. Some parasites, however, can establish inflammatory reactions in which malignancy can sometimes develop. These are rare in Western countries but are well known in other parts of the world; for example in Egypt a parasite that commonly lives in the bladder or bladder wall can predispose to the development of bladder cancer.

Hormonal changes

Some cancers are clearly related to circulating hormones, for example, breast cancer is more common in women who have a prolonged period of potential fertility, i.e. women who began to menstruate at a very young age and have a late menopause. Women who have their first child late in life or have never had a baby have a greater risk of breast cancer than women who have had babies early in life, possibly as teenagers. Women who took moderate doses of female hormones (oestrogens) to relieve postmenopausal symptoms were also found to be at a greater risk of breast cancer. Smaller doses still slightly increase the risk of breast cancer. Even very small doses of oestrogen hormones given to relieve postmenopausal symptoms may have some risk, but the risk is small and may be justified for women with severe symptoms, unless they are at special risk. Women at special risk, including those who have previously had a breast cancer and women from families with a high incidence of breast cancer, should avoid taking oestrogen.

Women living in countries where it is customary to have a diet rich in plant hormones, the phytoestrogens, have a lower risk of breast cancer, just as men on such a diet have a lower risk of prostate cancer. These relatively weak plant hormones seem to provide a counter-balance to the possible risk of over-production of stronger human hormones in some people of both sexes. The role of phytoestrogens in cancer prevention is discussed in Section 3, Simple diet.

Degenerations

All tissues change with increasing age but in some tissues, for example the exposed skin of the face, or the lining of the mouth, degeneration changes can be excessive and can lead to malignant change, i.e. cancer. There are a variety of causes of these excessive changes, for example repeated damage by sunlight, noxious irritants like tobacco, another disease process such as diabetes, chronic irritation or injury or low grade chronic infection.

The ageing process and ageing of tissues

The changes in tissues that occur gradually with ageing predispose virtually any tissue to increased risk of cancer. Some ageing tissues are more likely than others to develop pre-cancer changes in the nucleus of their cells; this explains the increasing risk of cancer in some tissues. For example, almost all men over the age of 90 have cells in their prostate glands that look malignant, even though not all of them will be growing or spreading in an aggressively malignant way.

There are a number of non-malignant (non-cancerous) conditions containing cells that have an increased risk of changing to become cancer cells. Amongst these are benign tumours. Benign tumours are local collections of a lump of cells in a tissue that look normal, or almost normal, and are usually surrounded by a capsule or membrane covering. This local collection of cells is not part of the normal body tissue and is not needed by the body. Benign tumours reach a certain size, then the cells stop growing and the tumour usually remains as a lump, unless it is removed or disturbed in some way. Examples are a lump of fat cells called a lipoma (these can occur anywhere in the body where there is fat), a collection of surface cells called a papilloma (a wart is an example), a lump of bone cells called an osteoma or a local lump of gland cells called an adenoma. While most benign tumours—for example warts—almost always remain benign and harmless, some do carry an increased risk of later developing into a cancer.

The beginning of a cancer

Whatever initiated the changes in cells—an inherited abnormality, chronic injury, chronic inflammation, exposure to a particular toxin or the ageing process—cancer begins when one or more of the many billions of cells in our body breaks free from its normal restraints and starts to multiply in an abnormal, uncontrolled and unrestrained way. This can happen to almost any type of cell; skin, gland, lining of mouth, throat, air or food passages or other passages or cavities, bone, fat, nerve, muscle or blood forming cells etc. Some are at greater risk of change than others depending on the cause, the patient's age, and many other factors, but once this unrestrained change in cells has become established it will continue. These cancer cells will cause damage to normal tissues and normal parts of the body unless the diseased area (the cancer) is removed or restrained or controlled in some other way.

Living conditions and surroundings (environment)

The air we breathe, smoke or toxins that we inhale, irradiation of skin or agents that come into contact with skin, irradiation of deeper tissues or organs, the food we eat (the presence of toxic ingredients in our diet or the absence of other essentials from our diet), and various chemical agents with which we might come into contact, may all at times have potential for starting tissue changes that could lead to cancer.

Genetic factors—oncogenes

All cells contain genes inherited from our parents. These genes are responsible for the reproduction of cells, maintenance of the different tissues and body functions, and normal body activities. Some genes are responsible for maintaining normal reproduction of cells in each tissue, either by stimulating cell reproduction or by stopping and limiting cell reproduction according to body needs. *Oncogenes* are those genes that are responsible for cancer cell growth. They may be inherited from a parent (i.e. congenitally abnormal genes) or may develop due to a mistake in the many billions of cells that reproduce for growth, development, and maintenance of tissue activity and tissue repair (i.e. they may be acquired from something causing a change in a normal gene). Such a mistake is called genetic mutation, and is most likely during the greatest activity and cell turnover of each body tissue. The wonder is not that some mistakes are made, but that more mistakes are not made over years of normal tissue growth, activity, maintenance and repair over many years. As we grow older, with so many new cells constantly developing in many tissues over many years, a mistake in cell reproduction leading to a cancer becomes more likely with each passing year. Hence most cancers become more common in older age groups.

It seems that the different cancer-causing factors, to be described in Section 3, change normal genes to become oncogenes that activate biological triggers in cells, stimulating the cells to reproduce indiscrimately and so become a cancer. Our best protection is to avoid such damaging agents (like tobacco) and to maintain good nutrition for normal cell reproduction and maintenance. We must also pay attention to cells or tissues that may be likely to change or may even have begun to change into an early cancer.

Cancer incidence

In white people, especially with a fair skin and living in sunny climates, skin cancers are by far the most common cancers. Most skin cancers are at least potentially avoidable, and if not avoided are usually readily detected and effectively treated with a low risk of fatality. This now includes the most aggressive of skin cancers, the melanoma.

Of the internal cancers in Western or developed countries, especially North America, the UK, northern Europe, Australia and New Zealand, prostate cancer is the most common in men and breast cancer the most common in women. Lung and bowel cancer are the cancers most common to both sexes. Of all cancers, lung cancer is the most dangerous. In America it now causes more cancer deaths than all prostate, breast and bowel cancers put together.

The table shows the American Cancer Society's incidence of the most common internal cancers for

Table 1 Incidence of the most common cancers, other than skin cancer

Cancer	Annual incidence	Deaths
Prostate (in men only)	198,100	31,500
Breast (almost all are in women)	193,700	40,600
Lung (in both sexes together)	169,500	157,400
Large bowel (in both sexes together) (colon and rectum)	135,400	56,700

the year 2001. The relative incidence in other Western countries is similar.

As the table shows, in the USA, lung cancer is the most common cancer in both sexes together. However, the relative index is slightly different in other Western countries. In the UK large bowel cancer and lung cancer are almost equally common, but in Australia and New Zealand large bowel cancer is more common than lung cancer. Despite this, in each of these countries lung cancer is responsible for most cancer deaths, simply because lung cancer is less often curable when diagnosed.

Section 3

Lifestyle practices to avoid, to change or to adopt

There are seven main actions for cancer prevention. Four of these we can take for ourselves: avoiding smoking, protecting skin from excessive sun or other UV light, following a simple good diet, and self-examination on a regular basis. The fifth involves screening for cancer in people at special risk, for which a combination of self-motivation, expert advice and government services is required. The sixth is surgery to remove any premalignant or potentially malignant lesions, and for this we must have medical advice and help. Finally the seventh, safe industrial practices, is largely the responsibility of our lawmakers.

The seven S's of cancer prevention

S for stop smoking and smoking-related activities;
S for skin protection against sun and solariums;

S for sensible diet;

S for self-examination;

S for screening and special tests in early cancer detection;

S for surgery to remove premalignant or potentially malignant lesions;

S for safe industrial practices.

S for smoking and tobacco or other smoking-related activities

The single most avoidable common cause of serious cancer is tobacco smoking. Tobacco contains a number of chemical constituents but has two dominant noxious ingredients, tars and nicotine. In the tar content there are many carcinogens (cancer-causing agents). The nicotine content is more responsible for heart and blood vessel diseases and the addictive properties that make the smoking habit so hard to quit. The best single rule is DON'T START SMOKING.

It is especially important to educate young people, by word and by example, not to start smoking. If they believe that taking preventive measures to avoid getting a cancer or other serious health problem in 10, 20 or 30 years time means worrying about old age, there are other messages relevant to their immediate well-being:

To more than half the population they are seen as doing something stupid and unattractive;

Their clothes and their breath smell repulsive to more than half the population;

They automatically become less attractive to more than half of the opposite sex, including those in their own age groups;

They start to look dirty and untidy, and like many smokers they are likely to develop unpleasant habits such as dropping cigarette ash, cigarette ends and empty packets;

They will soon develop a cough that will make them even less attractive;

The habit is expensive and the accumulated cost after a few years is substantial.

Like taking illicit drugs, smoking makes other people rich. It uses money that the smoker might otherwise spend on an overseas holiday or on other pleasurable and less dangerous activities: buying a nice car, paying a deposit on a home or just having a healthy savings account.

Apart from damaging their own health, if they have children, smokers run considerable risk of damaging the health and well-being of their children. Babies born of mothers who smoke are likely to be less healthy and more likely to be underweight when born. They are also more prone to problems like sudden infant death syndrome. Children living in a household where one or both parents smoke are more likely to have health problems, especially asthma and other respiratory problems, as well as an increased risk of some cancers later in life. They are less likely to grow as active, healthy children (Figures 1a and 1b).

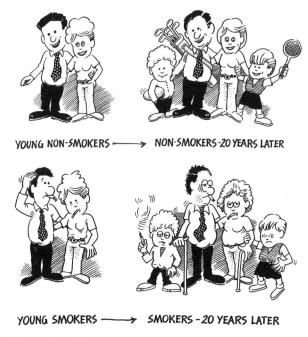

YOUNG NON-SMOKERS ──→ NON-SMOKERS-20 YEARS LATER

YOUNG SMOKERS ──→ SMOKERS -20 YEARS LATER

Figure 1 (a) Young non-smokers/non-smokers 20 years later; (b) Young smokers/smokers 20 years later.

Forms of tobacco taking and smoking

Taking tobacco products in any way has potential to cause cancer. Chewing tobacco causes cancer in the mouth and is even more toxic if the tobacco is mixed with lime or betel nut, as is the habit in some parts of India. Cigar smoking and pipe smoking are also associated with an increased risk of cancers in the lips, tongue and mouth. Passive smoking (breathing 'second hand' smoke in a smoke-filled room) or taking tobacco as snuff are also potentially carcinogenic. Cigarette smoking may cause any of the above mentioned mouth cancers as well as throat and larynx (voicebox) cancers and is responsible for lung cancer becoming the most common cause of cancer death in men during the twentieth century. In some countries, including the USA, it has also become the most common cause of cancer death in women. (The incidence in women is still increasing as greater numbers of women have been taking up smoking.) Cancers in the mouth, throat, and larynx are six times more likely to occur in smokers than in non-smokers, and cancers of the lung are about 10 times more likely to occur in smokers. There is also a significantly increased risk in 'passive smokers' i.e. people who live, work or closely associate with smokers but are not smokers themselves. There are also health problems in babies born to mothers who smoke and in children who live in a household with smokers.

Cancers of the mouth, throat, and larynx are often curable, but cure may involve partial or total removal of the tongue or the larynx (voicebox) leaving the patient unable to swallow or speak as others do. Cancer of the lung is not often curable and leads to a very unpleasant death.

Smoking can also cause emphysema, an incurable condition in which the small delicate air sacs in the lungs stretch or burst. Emphysema causes severe and choking breathlessness even at rest, and can be a protracted and unpleasant illness over a period of several years.

Alcohol and smoking

Evidence for alcohol being a direct cause of cancer is controversial; a more established association is evidence that alcohol seems to enhance the cancer-causing effects of smoking. Smokers have a six times greater risk of mouth and throat cancer than non-smokers; this increased risk is more than doubled if the smokers are also heavy drinkers of alcohol.

Cancers associated with tobacco smoking

There is an increased risk of many cancers associated with tobacco smoking. Lung cancer, lips, mouth, throat and larynx cancers are the most recognized, but others associated with the smoking include cancer of the pancreas (now the fourth or fifth most common cause of cancer death in males and fifth or sixth in females in Western societies), as well as cancers of the stomach, oesophagus, kidneys and bladder. The incidence of breast cancer is also increased in women who have smoked for 15 years or more, especially if they began smoking early in life before their breasts had fully developed. Recent studies have also shown that the risk of getting breast cancer is greater in women whose mothers were smokers or who lived in a house where one or both parents smoked. Although prostate cancer is probably not increased in numbers, the severity of the disease and the likelihood of fatality is increased in smokers.

Marijuana smoking

Like tobacco, marijuana contains a number of chemical agents with cancer-causing properties. Because marijuana is an illegal product it is difficult to make studies of the short and long term effects of marijuana use, even in Western countries where reliable health statistics would otherwise be available. Accurate figures on the exact risk of cancer are not available, but recent studies have reported that for equivalent amounts smoked, marijuana is at least as dangerous as tobacco.

There is a great deal of evidence of serious consequences of marijuana smoking including emotional and mental instability, problems with memory, concentration and learning ability and a loss of a sense of responsibility that can be particularly troublesome in driving motor vehicles or other machinery or in caring for children. There is also a loss of long term sexual prowess, increased fetal risks to unborn children, and an increased risk of lung cancer.

Recommendations

The most important rule for avoiding cancer is:
DON'T SMOKE.

Natural products

It is appropriate here to say a few words about 'natural products'. There is a tendency to assume that products grown or used in their natural states are good, and that anything altered chemically or developed in a scientific laboratory is automatically worthy of suspicion, if not contempt. This approach can be misleading. Tobacco and marijuana are 'natural' products, and some of the most powerful toxins and poisons are in natural plants or are products of plants. These include poison berries, poison leaves (e.g. oleander and rhubarb leaves), and poison mushrooms. Even strychnine is extracted from certain plant seeds. Of course it is true that many good and useful products used in medicine are also found in plants, including some herbs, and there are undoubtedly more valuable products to be discovered.

In some countries, such as India and New Guinea the betel nut—a natural product—is used as a pacifier. It is an inexpensive and habit-forming tranquillizer akin to tobacco, and like tobacco, it has carcinogenic properties. The custom in these countries is to chew the nut and then rest it in the cheek pouch until the next urge to chew it again. In many cases a fatal cancer will develop in the cheek pouch of the mouth after prolonged use.

S for skin protection against sun and solariums

The second of the major groups of controllable conditions in avoiding cancer is exposure to ultra-violet (UV) light. UV light comes primarily from the sun, but can also be experienced in solariums and is damaging from either source.

White-skinned Australians have the world's highest incidence of skin cancers and the incidence is also high in the southern United States. There are three major types of skin cancer: basal cell cancer (BCC), squamous cell cancer (SCC) and melanoma.

Cancers associated with UV light

Basal cell cancer (BCC)

The most common skin cancers are the basal cell cancers—and happily they have the lowest grade of malignancy. Basal cell cancers are slow-growing, very rarely spread to any other part of the body and are usually detected at an early stage, as they are easily seen on the skin when they are quite small. They are usually first noticed as a small persistent crusty lesion on the skin, as a small nodule in the skin or very often as a small painless ulcer that does not heal. These tumours can occur in the skin of any part of the body but are commonest in skin that is frequently exposed to sunshine, particularly the skin of the face. They are also common on the ears, the backs of the hands and forearms, and on the lower legs of people in sunny climates who wear shorts.

Squamous cell cancer (SCC)

Exposure to UV light rays also causes the second most common skin cancer—squamous cell cancer (SCC). These are more malignant than basal cell cancers; they tend to grow more rapidly and some-times spread to nearby lymph nodes or even to other parts of the body. Although skin is the most common site for SCCs, they can occur in other parts of the body where the lining cells of a hollow tube, for example the mouth and throat, the oesophagus, the vagina, or the anus, are like the lining cells of skin. However it is only in exposed skin that sunlight is responsible for squamous cell cancers.

Like the more common BCCs, these SCCs are seen most often in those areas of skin most exposed to sunlight. Both of these cancer types are uncommon in younger people, and tend to occur later in life in people more than 40 or 50 years of age, after an accumulation of years of exposure to the UV light of sunshine.

Melanoma and sunburn

The UV light of sunshine, or of solariums, is also responsible for the third most common but most dangerous form of skin cancer, the melanoma. Melanoma does not usually occur in places most constantly exposed to sunlight but in the skin of the back and chest, (especially in males) and the thighs and legs (especially in females)—skin normally covered by clothing. In contrast to the low-grade ongoing skin damage usually associated with BCCs and SCCs, the skin damage that predisposes to melanoma is not a gradual and daily repeated damage of constant or frequent exposure to sunlight but severe one-off, or severe occasional damage—the damage caused by sunburn. Melanoma most often occurs in an area of skin that has suffered sunburn in the past, especially if the sunburn occurred in childhood, often many years earlier. It seems that greatest damage is done to immune protective cells during early years of life, thus predisposing to an increased risk of melanoma developing later in life. Melanoma may develop at any age after the damage has been done, although onset before puberty is rare.

Recommendations

The important messages about the dangers of sunshine are threefold:

1. Avoid sunburn—particularly in childhood. Especially avoid the midday sun. Get children into the habit of wearing wide brimmed hats and other protective clothing, especially in sunny climates. (Some manufacturers now make especially protective light and cool clothing for this purpose.) If attending the beach or swimming pools do so in the early mornings or later afternoons and avoid the middle of the day, especially in summer. Wear a protective cream or lotion on any exposed skin (15+ is common but 30+ is better). The cream or lotion should be reapplied after each swim in the water. Adults should take similar precautions. Excessive or repeated exposure to the UV light of solariums is equally dangerous.

2. Avoid constant and repeated everyday exposure to direct sunlight at work or in sport or other outdoor activities. This is to avoid cumulative damage, especially to the skin of the face, ears, the head in balding people, the skin of the backs of the hands and arms, and other exposed skin such as the lower legs in those who wear shorts or short skirts. Fair-skinned people should get into the habit of wearing a wide-brimmed hat and wearing protective cream on the skin of the face, ears and other exposed parts. The lower lip and nose are especially vulnerable and often need extra protection, such as the thick layer of zinc cream commonly used by

cricketers and other sportsmen and women or workers exposed to long periods of sunlight. Some manufacturers now make women's face creams, lipsticks and other cosmetics with increased protective ingredients. These are recommended.

3. If any significant change is noticed in a brown, red or other localized spot in skin, or if a new and different spot arises and does not settle in 2–3 weeks, seek medical advice without further delay.

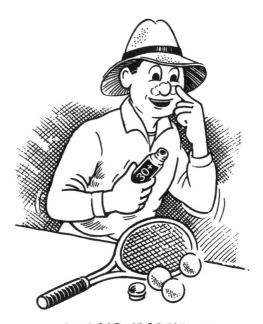

OUTDOOR SPORTSPERSON

Figure 2 Simple but effective measures to protect skin from excessive sunshine, particularly if taking part in out-doors activities. Note the hat, long-sleeved shirt, and protective sun cream.

Persistent crusty spots or ulcers may be cancers or may lead to cancers. A change in the colour or size or surface or appearance of a mole requires medical advice without undue delay.

S for simple diet

Soy positive—because soy is high in phytoestrogens and fibre.

Sausage negative—because sausages are high in animal fat.

The third of the major groups of important controllable conditions in avoiding cancer is to pay attention to diet. It has long been known that certain cancers—especially those of the digestive tract—can often be related to the food we eat or the food we don't eat.

Several specific cancers are associated with dietary factors to a greater or lesser degree. They include cancer of the stomach, large bowel, the pancreas, breast, and prostate. More will be written about these substances later in this book, but first something should be said about some cancers that have a special relationship to diet.

Cancer of the stomach

Stomach cancer has been associated with agents used in food preparation and processing and with specific food items. It is more common in men than women, and is one of the more serious and difficult cancers to cure. Fortunately it is becoming less prevalent, especially in Western societies. In early twentieth-century Western societies it was the second most common cause of cancer death in men and the third in women; in the last half of the twentieth century it became progressively less common. It is now about the eighth most common cause of cancer death in men and the tenth in women.

The reason for this decreasing incidence is not clear, although it is apparent that this cancer was much more common when chemical preservatives, especially nitrites and other salts, were routinely used in food preservation and storage. As refrigeration has become more widely available for food preservation and storage the incidence of stomach cancer has been decreasing.

In Japan, Korea and other Asian countries, stomach cancer is still very common although gradually declining. In Japan and Korea, strong spices and flavouring agents, salts and chemical preservatives are still used to flavour and preserve foods. In Korea the red chilli pepper is commonly used, and this has been found to be able to cause stomach cancer in animals when used in large amounts. Preservation of fish by smoking is still common practice both in Japan and Korea, and there is evidence that potential carcinogenic chemicals are produced by the smoking process.

Nowadays a diet with a higher content of fruit and vegetables, grains, fresh fish and more lean meat stored by refrigeration is associated with a lower incidence of stomach cancer than in those who eat diets with a high animal fat content or foods preserved by chemicals or by smoking.

Large bowel (colon and rectum) cancer

In some Western countries in the twentieth century (including Australia and New Zealand) the most common cancer of both sexes, apart from skin cancer, has been cancer of the large bowel. In the USA lung cancer is now more common but bowel cancer is second (see Table 1). The apparent reason for the high incidence of bowel cancer is the Western diet, which has a high content of refined foods with reduced quantities of natural roughage (fibre or glucan), vitamins and trace elements. Modern Western diets also have a much greater content of animal fats, including meats and dairy products, with a relatively low content of plant foods. Recently there has been a great deal of interest in the naturally occurring plant hormones *phytoestrogens*, and another naturally occuring component of tomatoes and some other red fruits and vegetables, an anti-oxidant called *lycopene*. These are a component of the diet of people living in less developed societies that have a lower incidence of certain cancers, including bowel cancer. These include African, Asian (except Japan), some Latin American and some Mediterranean countries.

Cancer of the pancreas

Pancreatic cancer presents as one of the most difficult and insidious of all cancers to diagnose and treat. It became increasingly common in both men and women, particularly in Western or developed societies, during the second half of the twentieth century. Many conceivable causes of this cancer have been widely investigated, but apart from a clear association with tobacco smoking there is little evidence to implicate any other single cause as being of major importance. It is more common in people with diabetes and in those with previous episodes of pancreatitis (inflammation of the pancreas). It is also more common in men than women, but why it has become more common in both sexes over recent years is not fully understood.

Cancer of the pancreas is more common in Western societies than in Asian countries, although the difference in incidence is not as obvious as it is for the other 'Western' cancers of the breast, prostate or bowel. There is some evidence that one reason for the increased incidence of pancreatic cancer might be reduced amounts of fibre and phytoestrogens or closely associated ingredients that have cancer protective properties. The difference in incidence is clouded by the close association of pancreas cancer with tobacco smoking. People who live in East Asian and South-East Asian countries with a high intake of phytoestrogens, fibre, vitamins, essential minerals, trace elements and anti-oxidants probably have some protection from their diets, much of which is lost due to the high incidence of tobacco smoking in many of those countries. Tobacco smoking is a highly significant factor in association with cancer of the pancreas but is of less significance in breast, prostate or colon cancer.

Breast cancer

Breast cancer, like bowel cancer, is sometimes called a 'Western disease'. Like bowel cancer it became more common in North America, the UK, northern Europe, Australia and New Zealand after the industrial revolution, when more affluent citizens became less dependent on large quantities of fruits, cereals, nuts, grains and vegetables, including legumes, and more dependent on fatty foods, meat and dairy products. Reduced amounts of the naturally occurring plant hormones, the phytoestrogens, and related compounds in modern Western diets as compared to the large amounts in vegetarian and Asian diets, is thought to be at least partly responsible for the increased incidence of breast cancer in women in Western societies.

As well as a higher intake of fruits and vegetables, women in some Mediterranean countries tend to have a relatively high consumption of lycopene in tomatoes and some have a daily intake of a glass or two of red wine. They also use polyunsaturated olive oil rather than saturated fats, especially animal fat. It is believed that these dietary differences may be responsible for the rather lower incidence of breast cancer in Mediterranean women compared to women of northern Europe.

Prostate cancer

Just as the incidence of breast cancer has been increasing in women of Western societies over recent decades with comparatively little increase in women of Asian or undeveloped countries, so too in men there has been an increasing incidence of prostate cancer in Western countries over about the same period. The incidence is greatest in the USA, Canada, Australia and New Zealand. Studies have shown that a likely related factor is the gradual changes in diet. In industrialized Western countries there has been an increased dependence on fatty foods, especially meats and dairy products, together with increased consumption of processed grains, refined sugars, and other refined foods. At the same time there was reduced consumption of fruits, vegetables, unprocessed grains and especially legumes like soya beans with a high content of the naturally occurring plant hormones, the phytoestrogens, and related compounds. Men living in Mediterranean countries also have a slightly lower incidence of prostate cancer than those of northern Europe. Again it has been suggested that the lycopene of tomatoes, a little red wine taken daily as is common practice, and the use of olive oil rather than animal fats in cooking may give some protection.

Traditional recommendations—a balanced diet

The traditional recommendation of nutritionists over the years has been to take a balanced diet. However, just what constitutes a 'balanced' diet varies in different societies and at different ages in the history of human evolution. For most of the twentieth century to most people in industrialized Western countries a balanced diet meant three good meals every day with basic ingredients of meat, eggs, full cream milk, white bread, cheese, butter, potato (often fried), green vegetables, a piece of fruit and a cake or biscuits. To the average Asian, a balanced diet would have meant rice and soy as basic ingredients, sometimes with fish, nuts, fruit and vegetables, and wholemeal or rye bread. This was closer to the diets of Westerners before the industrial revolution, when Westerners lived more simply and cheaply with more plant food and less animal products.

Simple diets

African, Asian and other similar diets are likely to include more roughage and fibre, more naturally occurring vitamins, minerals and trace elements, more naturally occurring plant hormones (the phytoestrogens) and less fat, especially animal fat.

A number of active components of phytoestrogens, called isoflavones, have been shown to have anti-cancer activity. These plant hormones are especially plentiful in soy and in all legumes, including the great variety of beans and peas. These compose a significant proportion of the diets of Asians and other communities with a low incidence of certain cancers, especially breast, prostate and colon cancer. Recent research has revealed that legumes also contain a range of other related compounds, some of which appear to have anti-cancer properties. These ingredients could explain the lower incidence of certain cancers in people who take diets high in soy and similar plant foods.

These diets and the everyday, inexpensive diets of some Mediterranean and Latin American countries especially, also have a high content of lycopene which is most readily absorbed from tomato pastes, tomato sauces and other forms of cooked tomatoes. One consequence is that certain health problems, especially of the bowel, some cancers, obesity, hypertension and some cardiovascular problems are less common in people who have lived and continue to live on these simple, predominantly plant food diets. The cancer benefits include less risk of cancers of the breast in women, prostate in men and bowel and possibly the pancreas in both sexes.

A number of vitamins and trace elements are also present in somewhat greater amounts in the diets of people who eat a lot of plant foods. These include especially vitamins A, C and E, the so called anti-oxidant vitamins. An as yet unproven but widely held belief of their special virtue is that anti-oxidants neutralize toxic radicals. Toxic radicals otherwise accumulate in tissues and the circulation, resulting from wear and tear of tissues or ingested in food or water supplies.

Studies to prove or disprove this theory are as yet incomplete, but many highly regarded dietitians and other food scientists hold the view that taking additional anti-oxidants may well be protective and can do no harm, provided they are not taken in excessive amounts. Vitamin A for example can be toxic, especially to skin, if taken in very large doses. The jury is still out on the matter of the value of additional anti-oxidants, but certainly the amounts in standard Western diets are low. A supplement to Western diets of these and some other trace elements and ingredients of plant food diets may well be of value, although this is not yet completely understood.

Selenium is another food ingredient widely held to have cancer protective value, especially in regard to gastro-intestinal, respiratory and prostate cancers. There is some animal and human evidence that selenium levels are low when these cancers are present, but there is uncertainty as to whether low levels of selenium helped cause the cancers or were a result of the cancers. Until this question is resolved it seems reasonable to supplement diets in places where selenium is in short supply in food. This includes food-producing areas in some parts of North America and Europe and much of Australia, due to low levels in the soil. However selenium is quite toxic if taken in excess, so any supplement to the diet must be carefully measured and administered at safe levels.

Recommendations from more recent studies

Apart from taking adequate amounts of certain vitamins and minerals and the need to avoid much animal fat or toxic food products, especially poorly preserved or chemically preserved foods, there has recently been a great deal of interest in the possible protective anti-cancer properties of four newly studied food contents. These are:

1. Natural fibre content, especially of fruits, vegetables, nuts, grains, mushrooms and other plant foods.

2. The natural plant hormones (the phytoestrogens) present in all plants and especially the types called isoflavones present in all legumes (bean and pea family plants).

3. The substance that is responsible for the natural red colour in tomatoes and red berries and some other plant foods. This is called *lycopene.*

4. The so called anti-oxidants, including vitamins A, C and E, that are believed to have a neutralizing effect on toxic products of tissue wear and tear, that is, tissue breakdown products in the body or of dietary intake of toxic products.

Summary and present dietary recommendations

It is probably impractical to suggest that all Westerners change their dietary habits to those of traditional Asian, Latin American, or undeveloped African countries, or even lower-risk Mediterranean countries, but some changes can be strongly recommended. These include less dependence on meat, especially fatty meat, dairy products, other sources of animal fat and refined foods, with a greater intake of fruits, nuts and vegetables with larger quantities of peas, beans or other legumes, more cooked tomatoes and more unrefined grains and cereals.

Possibly a more simple alternative would be to change the diet less radically but be sure to take adequate vitamins (especially the anti-oxidant vitamins A, C and E), certain naturally occurring minerals (a small amount of selenium may have some protective value) and an additional daily dose of the naturally occurring phytoestrogens and lycopene-containing foods like cooked tomatoes. Possibly a little red wine might also have some anti-cancer protective value. The most active phytoestrogens, the isoflavones, are now available in tablet, capsule or powder form. One product now available contains, in one small tablet,

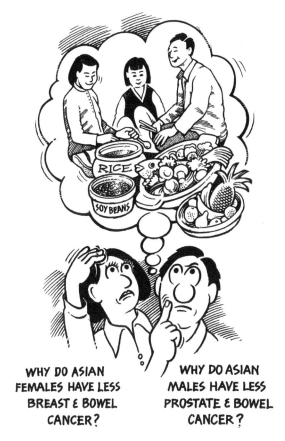

Figure 3   Why are people eating traditional Asian diets less likely to develop certain cancers?

a daily amount of phytoestrogens equivalent to that present in the diet of Asians who eat traditional diets with a high soy content. A similar product is made in Australia from the red clover plant, a legume with the richest known content of all the potentially helpful phytoestrogens.

'An apple a day keeps the cancer away' may be an over simplification, but there is some truth in it. Apples contain vitamins, fibre, phytoestrogens and anti-oxidants, especially in the skins. Other fruits and vegetables also contain at least some of these protective ingredients, but it should be understood that there is no quality in apples or anything else that will eliminate the harmful effects of tobacco or excessive smoking or other carcinogenic agents. Nor can any good product completely protect against the inevitable changes (genetic mutation) that take place with the turnover of many generations of cells over many years in the ageing process.

There is also evidence that the earlier in life good dietary habits are developed, the greater the advantage in reducing the risk of the 'Western cancers'.

S for self-examination

The fourth major group of controllable factors in avoiding cancers is to be vigilant in observing any unusual body changes and to seek medical advice if a possible problem is noticed. Such problems may range from lumps that can be felt in or under skin, change in a mole, an unusual discharge, bleeding from a duct or other abnormal spontaneous bleeding or change in bowel habits.

Simple precautionary measures carried out at home can help detect suspicious cancer lesions, especially in the form of breast lumps or skin cancers.

Breasts

Women are well advised to get into the habit of regular self-examination of their breasts. The best time to do this is once each month after menstruation has stopped and to continue a monthly examination after the menopause. The best place to do this is in the bath or under the shower when fingers are wet and soapy. Soapy fingers move more easily over the breasts and any lump is more easily felt.

Even if they were not intending to carry out a self-examination, most women who notice a lump in a breast first become aware of it when having a bath or a shower. There are a number of techniques or routines for self-examination of breasts, and it probably does not matter which is used as long as the woman is comfortable with it. The family doctor or a nurse in a breast clinic will give good advice if help is needed.

Skin

The other commonly practiced self-examination or family examination, especially for people at risk, is a regular skin check. People can usually see most of their own skin easily but it is good to have help of a partner or other family member or friend as a routine, perhaps every two or three months or so for examination of the skin of the back. This is recommended especially for people with a lot of moles, and particularly when they have a condition called *dysplastic naevus syndrome* with a lot of irregularly shaped, patchily coloured or large blotchy moles that sometimes run in families. It is also a good idea for anyone with a family history of melanoma or a previous history of melanoma themselves to have a regular routine examination of skin, especially for any change in a mole or a new mole or other unusual persistent skin lesion.

Testis

Although cancer of a testis is not common, when it does occur, it is most often in young men between 18 and 40 years of age. It is important to detect it early, because it is usually curable in its early stages and nowadays most are cured. Like all cancers, the earlier it is discovered the better the chance of cure, although with testis cancer the prospects of cure may still be good even in its more advanced stages.

Cancer of a testis is usually easily felt as a lump on a testis or sometimes as a more general swelling or enlargement of one testis. Most young men notice the lump or swelling themselves more or less by accident. Most lumps felt in the scrotum are not cancer, but some will be. However if young men take care to examine their testes at regular intervals, perhaps once a month or once every two months, they may detect a lump that could be an early and eminently curable cancer.

Bowel

Home testing for evidence of traces of blood in the bowel motion may well become routine in the future, especially for people with a family history or otherwise at special risk of bowel cancer. As yet a simple and reliable home test is not available in a generally acceptable form, but new test products are under study. A satisfactory testing product is sure to become available in the near future.

Blood, lumps, ulcer, pain

It must be emphasized that any unusual lump, bleeding, a persistent ulcer or unexplained pain or discomfort, especially if of recent origin, should indicate the need for medical advice. It should also be emphasized that not to seek medical attention because pain is not present with a lump or other abnormality might be missing the best chance of diagnosing and curing an early cancer. Pain is usually not a feature of cancer in its early stages.

S for screening for early detection and special tests in cancer detection

The best single precaution for patients wishing a check for detection and treatment of any potential cancer problem is a general examination by a family doctor. The doctor may well recommend one or more special cancer detection tests for people who might have a special risk.

In Western or 'developed' countries there are five organs or tissues that are commonly at risk of cancer development and for which some form of cancer screening test may show one or more suspicious lesions. The tests might reveal a lesion that could be either pre-cancerous and if treated possibly a cancer could be prevented, or show an early cancer not causing any symptoms but at a stage where given appropriate treatment a cure is highly likely.

The commonly used screening tests to screen for five of the more common potentially curable cancers are: the Pap smear for cancer of the cervix of the uterus; mammograms for breast cancer; prostate specific antigens (PSA) and digital rectal examination (DRE) for prostate cancer; occult blood and colonoscopy for bowel cancer; and skin cancer screening, especially the 'mole check' for melanoma and skin cancer.

Uterine cancer screening—the Pap smear test

The cervical smear or Pap smear is a test for cancer of the cervix of the uterus, and is probably the first and still one of the most useful screening tests. Cancer of the cervix is not uncommon, especially in women over 40 years of age who have had several babies. Incidence of this particular cancer rose in the latter part of the twentieth century as a result of the sexual revolution and the increase in the number of sex partners. The human papilloma virus is often transmitted during sexual intercourse and can predispose to development of cancer of the cervix. Development of cervical cancer is preceded by a stage where the cells covering the opening or cervix of the uterus undergo certain pre-cancerous changes. The Pap smear test is simple, painless and relatively reliable and can be carried out in a doctor's surgery. A swab or scraping of the opening of the uterus is taken through the vagina. Fluid from the swab or scraping is smeared over a glass slide and the cells on the slide are stained and examined under a microscope. Abnormal cells suggest that a cancer may be likely to develop, and appropriate treatment can prevent this. Sometimes actual cancer cells are seen and treatment at this stage should result in cure. An annual Pap smear test is often recommended, especially for women over 40 years of age.

Breast cancer screening—mammograms

Other than skin cancers, breast cancer is now the most common cancer in women of Western countries. Second is bowel cancer, then lung cancer but lung cancer has now passed breast cancer as the most common cause of cancer death in women in some Western countries including the USA and Canada. Screening clinics are now established in most major cities of Western countries and women at special risk, including all women over 50 years of age, are encouraged to attend at appropriate regular intervals for breast cancer screening.

Although there is no absolutely reliable screening test to establish a diagnosis of breast cancer, the most helpful non-invasive test is the mammogram. Non-invasive means that the test can be made without having to cut into or otherwise remove a piece of breast tissue. Mammograms involve taking special low dose X-ray films of the breasts. Cancer tissue can sometimes be seen in the X-ray films before the woman is aware of any problem and before any lump or other abnormality can be seen or felt. Cancer tissue appears rather more dense than normal breast tissue and often has very small spots of calcium in it—seen as tiny white spots in the X-ray film (see Figure 4c).

Lifestyle practices to avoid, to change or to adopt

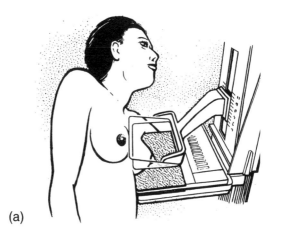

(a)

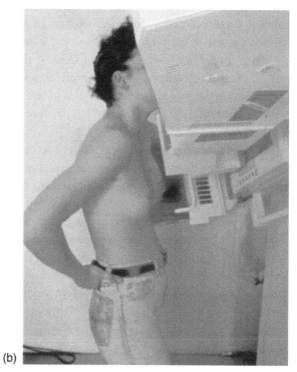

(b)

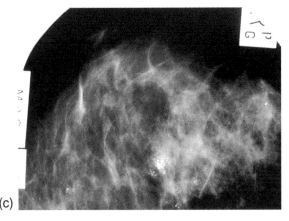

Figure 4   (a and b) A woman having a mammogram.
(c) A mammogram X-ray showing a small collection of tiny white spots that may indicate a cancer at that site.

Some women find mammography uncomfortable, because of the need to exert some pressure on the breasts as they are held between two plates while the X-rays are taken. The test is usually recommended only once every two years, or once a year in special cases. Given the substantial potential benefits, most women are prepared to accept a minute or two of some discomfort.

Doses of X-rays used are very small and in most cases can do no harm, provided they are not repeated too frequently. A mammogram every second year is usual for women over 45 or 50 but for women in special risk groups, such as a previous cancer in the other breast or a strong family history of cancer, it may be recommended that mammograms are scheduled more frequently or begin at a younger age.

Mammograms are not recommended during pregnancy or as a routine examination for women still in the reproductive age group, as even small doses of X-rays can be harmful to a fetus or to ovaries still making eggs (ovulating). For such women another non-invasive test, the ultrasound, may sometimes be recommended to help in cancer screening or testing of any small lump. The ultrasound may not be quite as helpful in diagnosing cancer, but it is a completely safe test in all circumstances, including during pregnancy. In younger women especially it is preferred to mammography, and usually shows lesions more clearly in the more dense breasts of young women.

No matter what these tests may show, a certain diagnosis cannot be made without a biopsy in which cells from the lump or a piece of tissue are taken for microscopic examination. These tests can sometimes reveal a very early cancer, often at a stage where it is premalignant or *in situ*, that is, when it is still a small collection of cancer cells in only one area of the breast. Such early *in situ* cancers are unlikely to have penetrated into nearby breast tissue or to have spread anywhere else and should be completely curable.

Prostate cancer screening—the PSA test and the DRE

Apart from the common skin cancers, prostate cancer is now the most common cancer affecting men in Western societies, but there is no highly reliable screening test available. The PSA (prostate specific antigens) blood test is now commonly used as a screening test in men over 50 or 55 years including those with no symptoms, although some doctors believe that this test should not be performed in men with no symptoms or no special risk of prostate cancer. A raised level of this test indicates some abnormality of the prostate gland. That abnormality might be cancer but is often just a benign enlargement of the prostate gland called *hyperplasia*. A raised PSA only suggests that further examination and testing for prostate cancer might be indicated. The PSA test is not totally reliable as the test index is often raised for reasons other than cancer in the prostate, and occasionally the test index is not raised even when a prostate cancer is present. Despite this, it is the best non-invasive prostate screening test available so far.

The other test for prostate cancer is a Digital Rectal Examination (DRE), in which a doctor feels the prostate with a gloved finger in the rectum. If the doctor feels a hard or lumpy prostate it may indicate a prostate cancer and should be further tested by a biopsy. A regular DRE every two years or so is recommended for Western men over 60 years of age or younger if there is a strong family history of prostate cancer. If there is a risk of prostate cancer it is best that both of these tests be carried out. A significantly raised PSA level might indicate that a prostate cancer is either present or might well develop within a few years. However, before a cancer can be diagnosed with certainty a biopsy of the prostate is necessary to provide microscopic evidence that cancer cells are present.

The main problem with any prostate screening test is that not all prostate cancers become invasive and behave aggressively, so not all men with prostate cancer may require active treatment. As yet there is no test that can indicate whether it will become invasive, spread to other tissues and need active treatment, or whether it would be better left alone because it will be unlikely to cause serious trouble during the patient's expected lifetime. Some doctors believe that until there is a test to determine whether a prostate cancer will become dangerous or not, it is better (i.e. kinder) not to do a PSA test in a man with no symptoms because a positive test may worry the patient unnecessarily.

Oesophagus and stomach cancer screening

Cancers of the lower end of the oesophagus and near the junction of the oesophagus and stomach are now becoming more common in many Western countries. Barrett's ulcer, which develops in the lower part of the oesophagus, can be a precursor of these cancers. People troubled with frequent reflux of gastric juices or food from the stomach into the oesophagus (sometimes known as severe heartburn) are most prone to a chronic, persistent inflammation—known as Barrett's oesophagus—in the lower oesophagus; some develop Barrett's ulcer. Chronic reflux can be treated by non-operative means or by surgery, but if the reflux or ulcer persist these sufferers should be kept under regular observation by screening with an endoscope (or gastroscope).

Bowel cancer screening (colon and rectum cancer)

Other than skin cancer, breast cancer is the most common cancer in Western women (followed by bowel and lung cancers). Prostate cancer is the most common internal cancer in Western men (again, followed by lung and bowel cancer). In both sexes together bowel (colon and rectum) and lung cancer are the most common, but lung cancer causes most deaths because it is not often detected at a curable stage. Lung cancer, being closely related to smoking, is common worldwide but breast, prostate and bowel cancer are known as the 'Western cancers'. Their high incidence is thought to be at least partly associated with the typical non-vegetarian diets of Westerners (see the section S for simple diet).

Screening tests for bowel cancer are now recommended more routinely for adults in Western countries in special risk groups. These include anyone with a history of bowel polyps or with a strong family history of polyps or bowel cancer. Some doctors, particularly in America, now recommend screening tests every two years for Western men and women over 50 years of age, especially if they are in a high risk group.

There are two main screening tests for bowel cancer. One is a test for the presence of blood in the faeces. This is called an *occult blood test* because the blood cannot be seen with the naked eye—occult simply means hidden. The other is for the patient to be examined with a special instrument, a colonoscope, which is inserted into the bowel through the anus. This procedure is called colonoscopy. A newer test, 'virtual colonoscopy', is being studied for its value and reliability.

The occult blood test is a chemical test done on a specimen of bowel motion. If persistently positive for blood it may indicate the presence of polyps; often these are premalignant and they should be removed to prevent cancer. A positive occult blood will sometimes indicate the presence of a cancer that has not been causing symptoms. Like most tests it is fairly reliable but not 100 per cent accurate.

Provided colonoscopy is carried out by a doctor who has had special training in using this instrument it should be a safe, painless and reliable procedure performed with the patient suitably sedated. The procedure is usually performed on an outpatient basis and the patient will only need to stay in hospital for a few hours. For most people, the doses of salts and excessive fluid that must be drunk to empty the bowel, often causing diarrhoea, are the only unpleasant parts of the procedure.

There are two more fairly common conditions of the large bowel that if not cured have a risk of developing cancer. These are a long-standing inflammation of the internal lining of the bowel wall—*ulcerative colitis*—and another rather different inflammatory condition of the bowel wall called *granular colitis* or Crohn's disease. After some years of uncured ulcerative colitis, removal of the diseased section of bowel may be advisable to prevent risk of cancer. Crohn's disease is less likely to develop a cancer.

Skin cancer screening—especially the mole check

Because there is a high incidence of skin cancers in fair-skinned people living in sunny climates, including a high risk of the most dangerous form of skin cancer, the melanoma, some clubs or workforces with members at risk routinely arrange special 'mole check' days. These checks have become increasingly popular in Australia, which has the world's highest incidence of these cancers. Australian Surf Clubs are foremost in using such facilities. Very often a mole or other pigmented skin lesion can be seen by an expert to have early malignant or premalignant features that threaten to develop into a fully malignant melanoma. Many lives have been saved by detecting and removing potentially threatening skin lesions before more serious or more advanced lesions have developed.

People who do not have an association with such a workforce or club may be well advised to have a regular check with their family doctor, especially if they have many largish or prominent moles or if there has been a family history of melanoma. If there is a special risk for someone with a lot of moles, or if they have dysplastic moles, the family doctor will often arrange an annual check in a specialist clinic (see S for self-examination).

Other screening procedures

Screening procedures for other cancers are some-times justified because of special needs. For example in Japan and Korea there is a very high incidence of stomach cancer, especially in males. A regular stomach examination with an endoscope is often recommended in those countries, particularly for males over 40 years of age. Tests for primary liver cancer are sometimes recommended as a regular routine in other countries where these cancers are common.

On the other hand in Western countries, lung cancer causes more deaths in both sexes together than any other cancer, but routine chest X-rays as screening tests for lung cancer are not commonly practiced. This is partly because of the need to stress the advisability of not smoking as the most effective preventative measure, but also because once a lung cancer can be seen in a chest X-ray the chances of it being curable are usually not good.

S for surgery to remove premalignant or potentially malignant lesions

Premalignant lesions are lesions that are likely to slowly progress and become cancer if left unchecked. *Potentially malignant lesions* are benign lesions that may always remain benign but have a greater potential to change than normal tissues.

For any of these conditions a doctor should be consulted.

Cancers are tumours or clumps of abnormal cells that continue to grow for no good reason. Cancer growth does not stop. It is not limited. The dividing cells are no longer under normal body control as regulated for body needs. Cancers get bigger and damage structures near them; also, they often spread to other parts of the body where they grow and damage other tissues and organs.

Benign tumours

Benign tumours are not cancers, but they also consist of abnormal collections of cells. Their abnormal

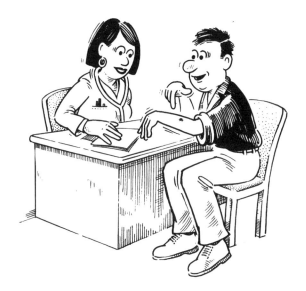

CONSULT YOUR DOCTOR

Figure 5   Anyone who notices something different appearing in the physical structure of their body (like a lump or a swelling or ulcer or discharge), or anyone who becomes aware of a new or different feeling or sensation (including pain but not necessarily pain) or a change in something (such as appetite or bowel habit or body weight or urine flow), should seek medical advice. This man has noticed a change in a mole in the skin in his forearm.

growth usually reaches a small size, then something causes them to stop growing. The cells in a benign tumour are essentially normal cells, but an excessive number of them have grown in the one place. It is not uncommon for people to have one or many benign tumours, that is, tumours that are not harmful. They are usually small, remain small and are some-times referred to as *innocent tumours* in contrast to the harmful or malignant tumour growths commonly called cancers.

Some benign tumours have a high risk of changing into malignant tumours (cancers) but with others the risk of becoming malignant is very small. Those that have a very low risk of changing into a cancer are usually left alone and treated only if a change takes place, for example if they start to get bigger. These include most small, usually soft fatty tumours called lipomas. Lipomas often occur under the skin but they can occur in any part of the body where there is fat. Firmer lumps called fibromas (consisting of fibrous cells) or neurofibromas (consisting of a mixture of nerve cells and fibrous cells) may also occur under the skin or in other places. Benign tumours also include small tumours of blood vessels that may look like red or pink lumps or patches in or under the skin—these are called haemangiomas.

For benign tumours with a high risk of becoming malignant (cancer) the risk can be avoided by removing them before any cancer changes take place. A doctor's advice should always be sought.

Common skin warts are another form of benign tumours of skin cells with virtually no risk of becoming malignant. However a different kind of wart-type lesion, caused by the human papilloma virus and sometimes sexually transmitted, does have a real risk of becoming a cancer.

Other benign (non-malignant) tumours that can become malignant

Any body tissue or organ can develop a benign tumour lump of apparently normal or near normal benign cells but in a local clump that is usually partly or completely surrounded by a capsule or fibrous sheath. These are not cancer but are benign tumours. They are benign because they seem to reach a certain size, often only about 1 or 2 centimetres in diameter, and then, unlike cancer, they stop growing. Also, unlike cancer, they do not spread to other parts of the body, they are not dangerous and are usually noticed quite by accident. But occasionally a previously benign tumour can change and become a malignant tumour or cancer. As malignant tumours they then continue to grow, expanding into and damaging the tissues around them. If they spread to other parts of the body and form new growing lumps, these are called secondary or *metastatic cancers* that then damage whatever tissues or organs they are growing in. Most benign tumours have little risk of changing into a cancer, i.e. becoming malignant, but some carry a greater risk.

Papillomas, adenomas and other
benign tumours

A benign tumour of surface lining cells is a papilloma; if it becomes malignant it is called a cancer or carcinoma. A benign tumour of gland cells is an adenoma; if it becomes malignant it is also called a cancer or carcinoma. However, benign tumours of other tissues are called by the Latin name of the cells in them. Thus a benign tumour of fat cells is a lipoma, of fibrous cells is a fibroma, of nerve cells is a neuroma, of muscle cells is a myoma, of cartilage is called a chondroma, and a benign tumour of bone is an osteoma. Cells of blood vessels can also form a benign tumour; these are called angioma or haemangioma if there is blood in them. If these types of connective tissue cells (i.e. non-glandular, non-lining cells) become malignant and behave like cancers they are technically known by another name—sarcoma. To all intents and purposes sarcomas are cancers but known by another name. Thus a cancer of fatty tissue is a liposarcoma, of fibrous tissue is a fibrosarcoma, of nerve tissue is a neurosarcoma, a cancer of bone is an osteosarcoma and so on. Any benign tumour can occasionally become malignant, so if a benign tumour shows any sign of getting bigger or otherwise changing it should be removed. Sometimes benign tumours are better removed whilst they are still quite small to prevent any risk of becoming malignant sometime later in life.

Benign tumours of glandular tissue are called adenomas. One or more adenomas can develop in the salivary glands (the largest is the parotid gland just below and in front of each ear), the thyroid gland (in the lower neck), the breast (or mammary gland), the ovary, the pancreas, the glands in the stomach lining or glands in the bowel wall. Benign adenomas often do not cause symptoms and are commonly found more or less by accident, but some can become malignant, and some types are more likely to do so than others. They should at least be tested by biopsy for malignant cells; even if they are found to be benign it may be better to have them surgically removed to avoid any risk of cancer developing.

Premalignant conditions responsible for some of
the more common cancers

Skin lesions

Some skin lesions are better treated or removed
before risking malignant change. These include
crusty lesions of the skin caused by repeated sun
damage—hyperkeratoses—and raised crusty horny
projections from the skin surface called cutaneous
horns. To prevent the more serious melanoma from
developing it is often advisable to have brown pigmented moles that have unusual features—dysplasia—surgically removed. (Dysplasia means an
irregular edge, irregular surface, or a mixture of light
and dark colour.) It is also usually advisable to have
any mole that has shown any change, especially a
mole that gets bigger or becomes itchy, or a mole or
other persistent skin spot that shows any change in
colour or change in the texture of its surface (e.g. a
flaky surface), surgically removed. If a mole is in a
position where it is likely to be constantly rubbed or
irritated, such as on the sole of the foot or under a belt
or bra strap, it may be wise to have it removed. A
mole that has become ulcerated is especially worrying.

Polyps—stomach, bowel etc.

These are benign tumours that are small lumps
mostly of gland cells (adenomas), covered by a thin
layer of surface lining but projecting from below the
surface of the lining of body cavities such as the
inside of the stomach or bowel. They look like
smooth lumps pushing up and under the surface lining, and will sometimes be attached to the tissue in

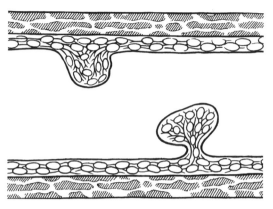

Figure 6 Polyps in the bowel. Polyps may simply be raised lumps under the lining of the bowel (sessile polyps) or they may project on a stalk into the bowel lumen (pedunculated polyps).

which they developed only by a thin stalk (Figure 6). Common places for polyps to occur include the lining of the inside of the nose, the lining inside the stomach or bowel or the lining of the cavity of the uterus or womb. They sometimes bleed and may cause bleeding from the stomach or bowel or vagina, or they may enlarge and cause obstruction to a passage such as the nose or the nasal passage (the air passage) behind the nose. In any case they are usually better removed to avoid any risk of malignant change taking place at a later date.

Some polyps have a very high risk of becoming malignant. There is an inherited condition of the large bowel called *familial polyposis coli* in which all people who have these polyps will develop a bowel cancer, usually before the age of 40. This is not common, but it is essential that all close relatives of a person with this condition are examined for polyps. Anyone found to have the polyps should have the large bowel (the colon and rectum) removed by a surgeon to prevent cancer developing.

Leukoplakia

Another group of premalignant lesions with a fairly high risk of malignant change which should be removed or otherwise treated include white plaques—called leukoplakia—in the lining of the mouth. They are most common in smokers, and can be the result of poor hygiene or poor cleanliness in the mouth, poor condition of teeth, or chronic irritation from excessive strong spirits, hot chillies or peppers, or other irritating spices. Leukoplakia is rather more likely to occur in diabetics and is occasionally the first sign of diabetes.

It can also occur in other places such as the vagina, but wherever leukoplakia is found it should be removed or otherwise treated to reduce the risk of a cancer developing. Any long-standing infection over months or years, especially fungus infection with the monilia fungus, can develop patches of leukoplakia either in the mouth or in the vagina, but often there is no obvious cause for the appearance of patches of leukoplakia.

Papilloma

A papilloma is a benign or non-malignant growth of surface cells. Like polyps some have a low risk of becoming malignant (like common warts), and others a high risk. A papilloma projects from a tissue surface, for example from skin or the lining of the mouth or throat or larynx (voicebox), or the inside lining of the bowel, kidney or bladder. A papilloma will sometimes develop in a duct, such as a milk duct of a breast.

As noted previously some papillomas are known to be caused by a virus, especially papillomas on the skin or lining of the vagina (see S for screening—uterine screening).

The common small warts and pigmented warts on skin are caused by a harmless virus but raised papillomas in skin are sometimes caused by a more troublesome virus, the human papilloma virus. The human papilloma virus can also cause papillomas in the lining of the vagina or cancers of the cervix of the uterus. Papillomas caused by the human papilloma virus are much more likely to become malignant (i.e. cancerous).

Papillomas look something like a very small fern or a very small cauliflower growing from the skin or another body surface. The risk of their becoming malignant varies from very small to moderate in most skin papillomas to a high risk in some bowel papillomas. Villous papilloma, which sometimes occurs in the large bowel, has many projections or fern-like leaves or fronds growing from the same patch of bowel wall (see Figure 7). This type of papilloma has a high risk of cancer developing and should be removed without unnecessary delay.

Recommendations

Some cancers can be avoided, by treating any pre-malignant condition or removing a benign tumour that has a risk of becoming malignant before any

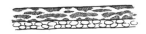
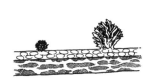
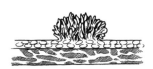

Figure 7   A small and a large papilloma projecting from the surface of skin. The diagram on the right illustrates a large villous papilloma which grows from the inner surface lining of the large bowel and is likely to develop into a cancer.

malignant change has taken place. Anyone who notices something different appearing in the physical structure of their body (like a lump, swelling, ulcer, or discharge) or anyone who becomes aware of a new or different feeling or sensation (for example in appetite, bowel habit, body weight, or urine flow) should seek medical advice. Medical advice should be sought about any such lump or change starting in a previously unchanged lesion, such as a mole, or any new or persistent abnormal discharge or bleeding.

It is also important to remember that pain is not an early feature of cancer. People who ignore a new lump or a change in a lump, or an ulcer, or unusual bleeding, or a change in a pigmented mole or other skin lesion, simply because it is not painful, may be missing their best chance of preventing or curing a cancer.

S for safe industrial practices

Some cancers are related to industrial practices and atomic, industrial or other forms of irradiation.

Industrial chemicals

Just as practices in other health areas have changed with accumulated experience and knowledge, so industrial legislation based on tragic early experiences has enforced protection against some cancers commonly seen in former years. One of these is a form of skin cancer of the scrotum, common in chimney sweeps of early industrial England. Soot from chimneys would collect in the trousers of these sweeps. Soot is now known to be an irritating carcinogen, and constant exposure over a long period could cause a cancer in the skin of the scrotum. The old practice of chimney sweeping without protection is now prevented by law and such cancers are no longer seen.

Another carcinogenic industrial practice of the nineteenth century—painting the dials and hands of luminous clocks with a phosphorus product—has also been outlawed. Workers would moisten the small brushes with saliva by putting them in their mouths. At each use a little phosphorus was absorbed and deposited in the bones; it accumulated and often stimulated a bone cancer.

In nineteenth-century Germany workers in aniline dye factories were found to develop a high incidence of bladder cancer from absorption of the dyes. Again, the unsafe practice of handling these dyes has long since been outlawed.

Asbestos

The association between lung cancer and exposure to asbestos has been well established, particularly if asbestos particles have been inhaled as asbestos dust. Asbestos is a fibrous material once commonly used in the building industry, and it is still present in many buildings. The risk is greater if people exposed to asbestos are also smokers. In addition to lung cancer asbestos can also cause mesothelioma, a cancer that most often develops in the lining around the lungs (the pleura) or sometimes in the lining of the abdominal cavity (the peritoneum). Strict industrial laws now control the use and handling of asbestos in most countries.

X-rays, gamma rays and atomic irradiation

Various experiences have demonstrated the suscepti-bility of human tissues to the cancer causing effects of penetrating irradiation.

Skin cancer was common in the hands of people who first used X-ray machines, who would hold the X-ray plates in their bare hands while X-rays were taken. Damage done by many repeated doses of X-irradiation is now known to be cumulative and carcinogenic. It is now forbidden for X-ray staff to hold the plates when X-rays are being taken.

Atomic irradiation from the bombs detonated at Hiroshima and Nagasaki, and more recently irradia-tion from the disastrous leak of radioactive material from the atomic energy plant at Chernobyl, caused a variety of cancers to develop in long term survivors. Most apparent were the increased numbers of people who developed leukaemias, but there were also increased numbers of people with several cancers of the skin, breast, and thyroid and sarcomas and lymphomas (cancers of lymph nodes or other lymphoid tissue such as the spleen or bone marrow).

Other forms of irradiation—microwaves, high tension wires, TV tubes, mobile telephones etc.

More recently there have been expressions of concern about the potential cancer risks of living close to high tension wires, or constantly being close to microwaves or television tubes. The possible risk of mobile telephones being held against the side of the head has also been under suspicion and is presently under serious investigation. Whilst possible risks of these sources of irradiation cannot be dismissed, there is as yet no conclusive evidence to substantiate or refute these anxieties. There is still a need for further investigation, but it can be said that if there is a risk it cannot be as obvious as the known dangers of carcinogens like tobacco.

Other toxins, carcinogens and dangerous irradiation

Industrial laws have long been in place to protect workers and citizens from known cancer-causing chemicals and other influences. These include protection against exposure to chemicals of petroleum and other industries, protection of workers against the problems discussed above—soots and tars, aniline dyes, asbestos and other carcinogenic chemicals— and protection against X-rays and other forms of commercial, scientific and technical irradiation. Hopefully international laws will protect us from the horrors of any further risk of atomic explosion, and strict and binding industrial practices will prevent any more Chernobyl-type disasters. However, national and international law makers must be constantly on guard and ready to react appropriately to any further knowledge of risks or potential risks in these areas.

Section 4

Specific cancers and practical individual measures to reduce their risk

This section is intended as a quick reference guide to specific cancers for readers who have a particular interest in preventing the risks of one particular kind of cancer. The risk of each of the following cancers can be significantly reduced by taking certain practical and precautionary measures. In some cases measures can be taken to reduce the risk of getting certain cancers, sometimes a very early cancer can be detected and eradicated before a more serious or dangerous phase has developed.

Skin cancers

The risk of most skin cancers can be significantly lessened by taking certain precautions:

Basal cell cancer (BCC) and squamous cell cancer (SCC)

The risk of developing these relatively common skin cancers can be greatly reduced by the following measures:

avoid excessive sun or UV light exposure from solariums or any other source, this applies particularly to fair-skinned people;

in sunny climates, for those who spend any time out of doors, the use of protective clothing—wearing broad brimmed hats, long sleeved shirts and possibly long trousers or long socks—is the first line of defence;

if some exposure is inevitable, application of 30+ sunscreen creams, lotions or ointments to exposed skin will reduce the risk of sunburn and sun damage to the skin;

application of the more protective zinc ointment may be recommended to the nose and lower lip if prolonged exposure is inevitable;

fair-skinned women exposed to sunlight should use skin creams, lipsticks and other cosmetics containing protective UV screening ingredients.

Early treatment is advised for any potentially malignant skin lesion, such as a crusty hyperkeratosis, a cutaneous papilloma, cutaneous horn or a persistent localized reddish patch known as Bowen's Disease. Skilled treatment of any small skin cancer is strongly advised before it has a chance to develop further.

Melanoma

Similar precautions to those listed above should be taken to protect the skin from sun damage, or damage from the UV light of solariums or any other source, but it is especially important to protect the skin of children and young people to avoid any sunburn.

Skilled medical attention should be sought at the first sign of any change in a mole or naevus. This is especially important if there is a change in size or pigmentation of a mole or similar skin lesion or a change in its surface to become crusty, flaky, brown or reddish or ulcerated or bleeding, or if a persistent itch develops in a mole.

Anyone with many largish or prominent moles, especially with a condition called *dysplastic naevus syndrome*, should be kept under regular medical observation. Dysplastic naevus syndrome is a type of skin with many flat moles that are sometimes quite large and may look like big blotchy freckles. They are often in the skin of the chest, abdomen, or back or on the thighs. They may have irregular brown pigmentation and an irregular outline. This skin condition sometimes runs in families, with a parent or one or more close relatives having the same type of flat or blotchy moles. There is a slightly increased risk of a melanoma developing in any one of these blotchy brown moles. People with this syndrome should be kept under regular observation, as should anyone who has previously been treated for melanoma or anyone who has a lot of moles, especially if they are large or dark or prominent or if there is a family history of melanoma. Also any mole or naevus in a position where it is constantly being irritated should either be removed surgically or at least closely and regularly observed.

Most fair-skinned people have some moles, so it is advisable for all of us to get into the habit of checking our moles ourselves on some occasions when we bath or dress. It is also a good idea to have a partner or friend or family member to occasionally check any moles on the back or other areas of skin not easily seen by ourselves. Wives are often the first to notice a change in a mole on their husband's back. Although melanoma in the hair of the scalp is uncommon, when it does occur, it is often a hairdresser or barber who first notices it.

It is important to appreciate that *pain is not an early feature of any cancer*. People who ignore a change because a skin lesion or a lump somewhere was not painful may be missing their best chance of having a cancer cured.

Lip, mouth and throat cancers

Like the nose the lips, especially the lower lip, are at greatest risk of being most exposed to the sun, so rules for skin protection especially apply to the lips. The lips are also at risk of damage from irritants like tobacco. Tobacco will affect not only the lips but also the lining of the mouth and throat.

Rules for reducing the risk of cancer in the lips, mouth and throat regions are:

avoid excessive sunshine on the lips, avoid smoking and avoid other chronic irritants or carcinogens like betel nut;

seek skilled medical attention for any persistent crusty lesion or persistent ulcer;

seek dental attention for any area in the mouth being constantly irritated by a jagged tooth or a denture;

seek medical attention for any persistent site of infection, any unusual lump or a papilloma-like projection from the lining of mouth or throat. Also seek attention for any prolonged change of voice or local irritation or unexplained bleeding from the mouth or throat.

Salivary gland cancers

These cancers are not common, but when they do occur it is usually as a lump in front of or below an ear, around the mouth area somewhere in the cheek, or under the jaw. There is no known way of preventing these cancers other than surgically removing any adenoma (benign tumour of gland tissue) or other benign lump in a salivary gland that can sometimes change into a cancer.

Thyroid gland cancers

Like cancers of the salivary glands, these cancers can sometimes develop from a pre-existing benign tumour. Any such apparently benign tumour, especially if it is one single lump, should be biopsied. If found to be an adenoma it should be surgically removed.

In some people, and especially in some parts of the world known as 'goitre belts', there may be a deficiency of iodine, an important ingredient for proper function of the thyroid gland. Iodine deficiency can lead to cysts and other changes in the thyroid gland, and occasionally a cancer will develop in such a thyroid. An effective treatment, often carried out by health authorities in goitre belt regions, is to ensure that people likely to be affected are given additional iodine. This is often provided as iodine added to all salt sold in shops or otherwise used in the region. For those who do not add salt to their foods, some other means of taking additional iodine is recommended, partly as a cancer-preventive measure. The flesh of fish is a good source of iodine, thus people who eat a lot of fish are not likely to develop a goitre.

Oesophagus cancer

The oesophagus (in America spelt 'esophagus') is the tube that passes through the chest for passage of food from the mouth to the stomach. Cancers of the oesophagus have not been common in Western countries, but they are common in Asian and some African countries where food is often contaminated with organisms or a fungus or preserved with chemical preservatives. Cancer of the oesophagus is also more common in smokers.

However, cancer of the lower end of the oesophagus is now becoming more common in Western countries because it can develop in an inflamed and irritated lower oesophagus—Barrett's oesophagus—in which Barrett's ulcer sometimes develops (see Section 3). The irritation of Barrett's oesophagus and Barrett's ulcer are caused by stomach contents regurgitating or refluxing into the oesophagus, and this has become more common in Western countries for reasons not completely understood. Apart from avoiding eating contaminated foods and not smoking, the best precaution is to seek medical attention if food or gastric juice constantly regurgitates or if you are experiencing constant pain or discomfort behind the breast bone (the sternum).

The first evidence of oesophageal cancer is often a sensation of food getting stuck in the chest behind the breast bone after swallowing. Anyone with this problem should seek medical attention without delay.

Stomach cancer

Apart from not smoking, the risk of this cancer is best reduced by keeping to a diet of fresh foods, predominantly fresh fruits and vegetables, and avoiding chemically preserved foods. A high content of fatty foods or smoked foods and a high content of especially irritating foods like the red chilli or pepper should also be avoided. Another precaution is to have any premalignant lesions treated, such as stomach polyps or a long-standing stomach ulcer. (Polyps may cause bleeding and ulcers cause long-standing stomach pain and discomfort.)

In Japan and Korea, where stomach cancer is common, especially in middle aged and older men, regular screening examination of the inside of the stomach by an endoscope (an instrument passed through the mouth) is sometimes recommended. This is most often advised for men over 40 years of age, and results of treatment are much better if small cancers are detected and treated early in the disease.

In Western countries cancer of the lower end of the oesophagus and upper end of the stomach are now becoming more common, so regular screening by endoscopic examination is now recommended for people troubled with persistent and uncontrolled gastric reflux. Since the discovery and treatment of the ulcer-causing organism, *Helicobacter pylori*, cancers of the lower part of the stomach have become less common. The increasing risk of cancer of the upper stomach or lower oesophagus is predominantly in people with regurgitation causing chronic inflammation or ulceration known as Barrett's oesophagus or Barrett's ulcer. This condition should be treated either by conservative (i.e. non-operative) means or sometimes by a surgical operation to prevent the reflux.

Large bowel (colon and rectum) cancer

Large bowel and lung cancers are now the internal cancers most common to both sexes together in some Western countries including Australia and New Zealand (see Table 1). As described in the section on diet, the risk of large bowel cancer can be significantly reduced by keeping to diets that consist predominantly of plant foods, including fresh fruits, vegetables, nuts, cereals, grains and especially legumes. Fatty foods and large quantities of meats and dairy products are best avoided. Wholegrain, wholemeal or rye bread, wholegrain flour and other high fibre foods should be a standard part of the regular diet but highly refined foods like sweets, sugar, cakes, biscuits or white bread should not be a major part of the regular diet.

Polyps of the colon or rectum should be removed. They often cause bowel bleeding with blood in the faeces, and can now be removed by a skilled doctor using a colonoscope passed through the anus. Anyone who has had polyps should have regular follow-up examinations, possibly on an annual basis. It is also advisable that regular colonoscopic examination be carried out on close relatives of anyone who has had a bowel cancer or who has a family history of polyposis (many polyps). Given the high incidence of colon and rectum cancer in Western countries some doctors recommend regular colonoscopic examination, perhaps every two or three years, for all people over 50 years of age.

In recent years a small daily dose of aspirin has been used to 'thin the blood' in people who have suffered heart or blood vessel blockage problems. A very small dose of aspirin is effective in reducing blood clotting tendencies. It has recently been shown that a small dose of aspirin taken daily also reduces the risk of bowel cancer. It seems that, unless there is some contraindication to it, people over 40 years of age who continue to adhere to traditional Western diets might be well advised to take this small amount of aspirin daily.

Chronic inflammatory conditions in the large bowel may also predispose to bowel cancer. The condition known as ulcerative colitis is especially prone to cancer development if it has been present for ten years or more. If it cannot be cured or controlled, and especially if a long section of the bowel is affected, consideration should be given to having that part of the bowel removed surgically.

Another type of persistent and often recurrent chronic inflammation that is fairly common in large bowel—granular colitis or Crohn's disease—is less likely to develop malignant change, although it may do so if not well controlled over a period of years.

Gall bladder cancer

Cancers of the gall bladder are unusual in Western countries but are much more common in other parts of the world, including some parts of India. In the Western world this cancer has usually developed in a gall bladder that has been irritated by the presence of gallstones for several years. Occasionally when a gall bladder has been removed for stones, an unsuspected cancer may be found in the gall bladder wall. When a gall bladder cancer is large enough to cause pain, discomfort, jaundice or other symptoms it is usually quite advanced and unlikely to be curable. This is one reason why it may be considered advisable for a surgeon to remove a gall bladder from anyone known to have gallstones for a long time, even if the stones are not causing symptoms, particularly if the patient concerned is young and with an otherwise long life expectancy.

Cancer of the pancreas

The single most significant known cause of pancreas cancer is tobacco smoking. Without any doubt smoking should be avoided. However, as discussed in the section on diet, there is also evidence that diet may also play a role in this cancer. The evidence is not yet certain, but in order to reduce the risk of getting this cancer people are well advised to refrain from smoking and to keep predominantly to a diet of plant foods with a high content of fresh fruits and vegetables, nuts, grains, unprocessed and unrefined foods containing fibre, roughage, adequate vitamins, trace elements and minerals and other naturally occurring plant ingredients. Dietary fibre is probably protective but the role of phytoestrogens and related compounds, especially present in soy and other legumes, is still uncertain. However, evidence suggests that phytoestrogens may have protective properties against pancreas cancer as well as several other cancers. Other food and drink products that have been well studied in relation to pancreas cancer include alcoholic drinks, coffee and tea. The most commonly suggested associations are that alcohol and coffee in large amounts may have some detrimental effect with some increase in cancer risk, but tea might have a small protective advantage, possibly due to its antioxidant content. As yet evidence of their effects on the risk of this cancer is still unproven, somewhat controversial and probably not of a high order of magnitude.

Other widely studied associations of pancreas cancer are diabetes and pancreatitis, but it is still uncertain as to whether these conditions might cause the cancer or may sometimes be the result of a previously undetected underlying cancer. In any case, these conditions should be treated on their own merits.

Liver cancer

There are two main sorts of liver cancer—primary and secondary (or metastatic).

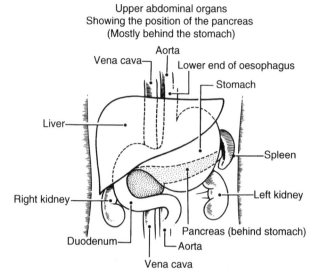

Upper abdominal organs
Showing the position of the pancreas
(Mostly behind the stomach)

Figure 8 The position of the organs in the upper abdomen. The pancreas, lying across the posterior wall of the abdomen, behind the stomach, and extending from the spleen on the left side to the duodenum on the right, is perhaps the least known organ, yet it is one of the more common organs for developing a cancer.

Primary liver cancer (hepatoma) is a cancer of the liver cells; that is, the cancer starts in the liver itself. This is often, at least theoretically, an avoidable cancer. It is common in countries and communities where hepatitis is common, especially hepatitis B and hepatitis C. These hepatitis infections are caused by viruses that are commonly present in South-East Asia and parts of Africa. The viruses are often transmitted by food, by sexual contact or by other close contact. Best protection is by avoiding such close contacts and meticulous cleanliness, especially in the preparation and handling of food. Protection against the hepatitis B virus can be achieved by immunization and this is recommended for people at special risk, especially those travelling to Asia or Africa. As yet there is no effective immunization against the hepatitis C virus.

Another association with hepatoma is cirrhosis of the liver. In Western countries cirrhosis is often caused by excessive and long term alcohol intake and alcoholics are at increased risk of these cancers.

Secondary liver cancer is one that started as a primary cancer in some other part of the body and has spread to the liver. Cancers starting in almost any tissue or organ in almost any site can sometimes spread through the blood stream to the liver and grow there. These can be avoided only by successfully treating and eradicating the primary cancer, wherever it is, before it has spread. Cancers of the stomach, the pancreas and the bowel most commonly spread to the liver. The liver is also a common place for secondary spread (metastasis) of advanced breast cancer and advanced melanoma.

Lung cancer

Of all of the cancers associated with cigarette smoking, lung cancer is the most obvious. It is common in all countries and communities where smoking is common, and the increased incidence during the twentieth century has been directly related to the increased use of tobacco. At first lung cancer was more common in men, but since more women took up smoking an increased number of cases are now being seen in women. In general the increase in lung cancers starts to become apparent about 20 years after starting smoking.

Lung cancer has been the most common cause of cancer death in men for more than 40 years, and in some Western countries it has now become the most common cause of cancer death in women. It is also a fact that smokers are about 10 times more likely to get a lung cancer than non-smokers. It is therefore clear that the single most effective precaution people can take to avoid a cancer death is NOT TO SMOKE.

Other possible causes of lung cancer include inhalation of noxious fumes from motor cars and other chemical products, but any risk of these associations is small in comparison to the risk of tobacco smoke, whether taken directly by smokers or indirectly by passive smoking. Industrial laws protect workers from possible exposure to industrial contaminants, but in most countries legislation has been slow to protect people against tobacco smoke.

As discussed in the section on smoking, evidence is less clear about the risk of smoking marijuana. It seems that the marijuana risk of lung cancer is similar to the risk with tobacco, but of course there are also a number of other risks with both products.

Breast cancer

Cancer of the breast is the most common among women in most Western countries, but in some countries, including some parts of the USA, lung cancer is now almost as common. In some Western countries lung cancer has become the most common cause of cancer death in women, but breast cancer remains either the first or second most common.

Breast cancer became increasingly common during the twentieth century, although latest figures indicate that the increase reached a plateau in the 1990s and may now have passed its peak. It may even have started to decline. It is to be hoped that the present suggestion of a decline in incidence will continue.

Although the exact cause or causes are not clear, a number of risk associations are known with breast cancer. For example, women who have their first baby as teenagers have a lower risk than women who have never had a baby or had their first baby when over the age of 35. Women who breastfeed their babies may also have some further protection. These are largely social events that cannot easily be changed. There is an increased risk of breast cancer in close relatives of women who have had a breast cancer. A very high increase in some families carrying a high risk gene is sometimes seen, but this is not common.

For premenopausal women at increased risk removal of the ovaries will reduce the risk, but this is usually not an acceptable solution.

The anti-oestrogen drug, tamoxifen, will reduce the risk of developing breast cancer and is recommended for women in high risk groups, such as those who have already had one breast cancer or women in families with a high risk. However women keen to have another baby are not given tamoxifen. Tamoxifen will reduce the risk of breast cancer but further studies are needed to find out whether, in women without any particular high risk, the likely benefits of tamoxifen are justified in view of possible long term side effects (e.g. slightly increased risk of uterine cancer). As yet there is no totally reliable preventive solution other than removal of both breasts early in life, and such an extreme measure is not an acceptable general solution. Workers in genetic engineering may provide a more acceptable solution in the not too distant future. BR-CA (BR from BReast and CA from CAncer) genes have been discovered in some women with breast cancer and are known to be associated with a higher risk of breast cancer.

Occasionally a premalignant condition can be detected and dealt with to avoid a cancer developing. One of these is a papilloma that may first cause a little discharge or bleeding from a nipple. However, the most accepted precautionary measure is breast screening of women over 40 or 45 years of age by use of mammograms, perhaps every two years in the first instance, and possibly the use of other special tests such as ultrasound studies in cases where doubt exists, especially in younger women. Biopsies should be taken of any suspicious lesion. These tests do not prevent cancer, but they do help detect early cancer at a stage when it can be treated most simply and effectively.

In recent years a great deal of consideration has been given to the possibility of reducing the risk of breast cancer by paying special attention to diet. As discussed in the section 'S for simple diet', there is a lower incidence of breast cancer in women in some countries, especially in Asia, Latin America, most of

Africa and even some Mediterranean countries. There are several possible reasons for this, including the custom of having children early in life. Another important reason appears to be the traditional diets of those countries and communities. In fact when African or Asian women live in Western countries and adopt Western habits and customs, including Western diets, or when Asian women in Singapore and Hong Kong live in a Western style, their risk of breast cancer is similar to the risk in Caucasian (white) women of their adopted countries. It seems apparent that the ingredients of their diets are significant in changing the risk of breast cancer. There is evidence that one of the special protective ingredients of the diets of Asians and other women with a low risk of breast cancer is the large quantity of the natural plant oestrogens called phytoestrogens. These agents are present in all foods of plant origin and are especially plentiful in all legumes, particularly soya beans, although the red clover plant has been found to be the richest source. Soy, which has a high content of the isoflavone type of phytoestrogens, is a traditional part of Asian diets. Soya beans provide an inexpensive form of protein as well as carbohydrates, vitamins and other essential ingredients, but little fat. Modern Western diets are based on meat and dairy products that contain much animal fat but no phytoestrogens.

A practical consideration for women wanting to reduce their risk of breast cancer therefore could be to adopt a change of diet from one based on meat, animal fat, refined foods and dairy products to a diet rich in unprocessed foods of plant origin and especially soy and similar legumes. There is also evidence that to have a major influence these dietary habits are best adopted at a young age, and are likely to be less effective if the changes are made later in life.

If major changes in dietary practices are not acceptable, a viable alternative would be to modify Western diets by reducing the content of animal and dairy products, especially their animal fat content, but supplementing it with increased plant foods and fibre containing foods. Taking a daily tablet of a preparation of phytoestrogens now commercially available might also be protective. As mentioned in the section on diet, the legume red clover has been found to be the richest source known of the whole range of phytoestrogens. Current investigations show that the red clover plant contains not only the full range of phytoestrogens but also some other related compounds that appear may also have potential anti-cancer properties.

After menopause women are sometimes prescribed small doses of oestrogens to relieve hot flushes, osteoporosis and a variety and range of distressing post-menopausal problems. Oestrogens in women of this age group do have a slight risk of increased stimulation of breast cancer. Studies are presently being made to discover whether phytoestrogens, being naturally occurring plant hormones and less stimulating than human oestrogens, might be effective in relieving these postmenopausal symptoms without the problem of increasing cancer risk to the breast. Results of these studies are not yet complete.

A more recently studied association of diet and breast cancer has been based on the lower incidence of breast cancer in the women of some Southern European and Mediterranean countries compared to northern Europeans, North Americans, Australians and New Zealanders. In Mediterranean countries, women who drink a little red wine daily and have diets containing relatively large amounts of tomatoes (such as pizzas and other foods containing tomato paste etc.) and use olive oil in preference to animal fat in their foods, do have a lower incidence of breast cancer.

Evidence now suggests that the red colouring ingredient lycopene, found in several plant foods but especially in tomatoes, may be at least partly protective. It has also been reported that lycopene is more readily absorbed from food containing cooked tomatoes, including tomato sauces or tomato pastes, than from fresh tomatoes. This might be good news for those who like to smother their food with tomato sauces or tomato pastes!

Cancers of the uterus

There are two types of cancer of the uterus, cancer of the cervix (the entrance of the uterus) and cancer of the body (the lining of the cavity of the uterus).

The cervix of the uterus

Uterine cervix cancer is the more common; although it occurs most often in middle-aged women it can occur in younger women. It is also rather more common in women who have had several babies. This is possibly due to damage to the cervix of the uterus with repeated childbirths. Cancer of the cervix is also more common in women who have had multiple

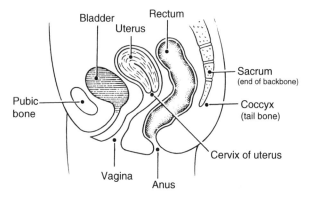

Female pelvis showing the position of
female genital organs. The ovaries are on
either side of the uterus

Figure 9 The organs in the female pelvis. The cervix, or
entrance of the uterus, is the most common site of cancer in a
woman's pelvis. To some extent this is an avoidable cancer,
but it is also the cancer most likely to be detected at an early
and curable stage by the Pap smear.

sex partners. Prostitutes are at special risk; one
reason for this is a greater risk of exposure to the
sexually transmitted human papilloma virus. This
virus is now a well recognized cause of cancer of
the cervix. Recent attempts to develop an effective
vaccine are showing some success.

Cancer of the cervix can usually be detected in its
earliest phase by the Pap smear (the Papanicolaou
screening test). This excellent test will usually
indicate the presence of any abnormal cells likely
to become malignant or the presence of actual malignant cells, so that appropriate prevention or treatment can be planned without further delay. All
women who have been sexually active but especially

women who have had a damaged cervix from previous pregnancies or women otherwise at special risk should have the test at regular intervals. A test once a year is usually recommended so that any area with abnormal cells that could become cancer can be treated, or if early cancer is detected it can be treated at a curable stage.

Another association with cancer of the cervix is the human papilloma virus. This virus predisposes to cancer of the cervix in some women and is commonly transmitted in the act of sexual intercourse. It is probably the most significant reason why women who have had a number of sexual partners are more at risk of being infected and subsequently at greater risk of getting cancer of the cervix. Recent attempts to develop an effective vaccine against human papilloma virus are showing some signs of success and a vaccine is now feasible.

The body of the uterus

Cancer of the body of the uterus more commonly occurs in women of older age groups. It often causes bleeding or vaginal discharge and is best detected by pelvic examination and curettage. Occasionally it develops from a polyp that might also cause vaginal bleeding or discharge, so that removal of a polyp may sometimes prevent a cancer from developing. This cancer is a little more common in women who take long term anti-oestrogen (tamoxifen) as treatment or for prevention of breast cancer. Women on long-term tamoxifen treatment should therefore have regular gynaecological examinations to detect and treat any early evidence of this cancer. Studies are in progress to determine whether the naturally occurring plant oestrogens, the phytoestrogens, might be effective if used instead of tamoxifen to give protection against breast cancer. If so it may be possible to give protection without the risk of stimulating cancer of the uterus.

Cancers of the ovary

With changes in the menstrual cycle small naturally occurring physiological cysts come and go on the ovaries, but sometimes a larger lump develops on one ovary and persists. It may cause some pain or discomfort, or may not cause any symptoms but simply be found at a general examination for something else. The majority of such ovarian lumps are either simple benign cysts, adenomas or other simple benign lumps (sometimes a mixture of benign adenoma and cysts). However, cancers do sometimes develop either from ovarian tissue or from a pre-existing cyst, adenoma, or other lump. Other than by removing both ovaries (generally not acceptable, especially to younger women), the only really effective way of reducing this risk is to surgically remove any known cyst of more than a few centimetres diameter. If such a cyst is persistent and still present at a repeated examination in a month or so, its removal should be considered.

Prostate cancer

Just as breast cancer is unusual in Asian and African women living on their traditional predominantly vegetarian diets but is common in these same people living in Western communities and having Western diets, so too the incidence of prostate cancer in men appears to be related to the dietary habits of their communities.

Like breast cancer in women, prostate cancer in men of the same Western communities became more common during the twentieth century. As with the incidence of breast cancer, it does seem that prostate cancer may have reached its peak incidence in the late twentieth century. Like breast cancer in women, prostate cancer in men is often hormone related and men having diets rich in plant hormones, the phytoestrogens, do have a lower risk of developing this cancer.

There is evidence, therefore, that men wishing to reduce their risk of prostate cancer would do well to consider changing from a traditional Western diet, based largely on meat and dairy products with a high animal fat content, to diets based predominantly on plant foods. Such a diet should contain plant foods with a high content of phytoestrogens and related compounds; thus larger quantities of legumes like soya beans are to be recommended.

For those not prepared to make major changes in diet, consideration can be given to following a diet with reduced animal fat content and supplementing this with a daily tablet of a commercially available phytoestrogen preparation. As yet there is no proof that these dietary measures would reduce the risk of prostate cancer, but circumstantial evidence suggests that there could be benefit.

As for breast cancer in women, recent studies suggest that a lower incidence of prostate cancer in men of Mediterranean countries might also be related to the red colouring ingredient lycopene, present in certain foods, especially tomatoes and red berries. Red wine also seems to have a similar protective value. Studies are not yet complete but there is evidence that men who eat a lot of cooked tomatoes (for example in pizzas, tomato sauces, and tomato pastes) and men who drink a little red wine daily and eat food containing olive oil rather than animal fat, have been found to be at lower risk of prostate

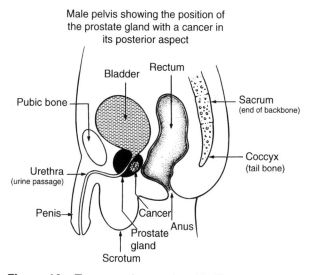

Male pelvis showing the position of the prostate gland with a cancer in its posterior aspect

Figure 10 The organs in a man's pelvis. The prostate gland is perhaps the least understood by most people, yet it is the internal organ that most commonly develops a cancer in men. The prostate gland is deep in the pelvis, behind the pubic bone, under the bladder, and in front of the rectum. The illustration shows a typical site of a cancer in the prostate gland. A doctor, with a gloved finger in the rectum, can often feel a prostate cancer as a hard prostate or a hard lump in the prostate.

cancer than British, northern European, North American, Australian or New Zealand males.

For many men, a diet containing pizzas and tomato pastes, a little red wine daily and a recommendation of smothering food with tomato sauce will be more than acceptable as a dietary recommendation!

Cancers of the testis

These cancers are not common, but when they do occur it is usually in young men between 18 and 40 years of age. One congenital abnormality of the testis—an undescended testis—has a high risk of becoming malignant, and early treatment can greatly reduce this possibility. In fetal life the testes develop in the fetus's abdomen but should descend into the scrotum before birth. Occasionally one or both testes fail to descend and cannot be found at birth or in early infancy. The testis will be present somewhere, either still in the baby's abdomen or somewhere between his abdomen and his scrotum. Such a testis has a high risk of becoming malignant later in life unless surgically brought down in childhood (by about 8 years of age) and anchored in the scrotum. Alternatively it should be surgically removed to avoid the risk of a cancer developing in adult life.

Kidney and bladder cancers

The most significant preventive measure adults in Western countries can take to help avoid kidney and bladder cancers is not to smoke. One other measure is to have any pre-cancerous lesions treated by appropriate experts. The most common of these are papillomas that occur especially in the bladder; they sometimes bleed and cause blood in the urine. These papillomas are often small and multiple, and can often be kept under good control and malignancy avoided by cautery (burning) done by a specialist urologist using an instrument passed through the penis and urethra—the passage for urine—into the bladder. This procedure may have to be repeated on several occasions, possibly twice a year. Another occasional cancer prevention measure is to remove any irritating stones from the kidney or bladder. In countries like Egypt where parasite infestation of the bladder is common, precautions taken to avoid bladder parasites will also help avoid the risk of a cancer.

Section 5

Conclusions

Cancer is a dreaded disease. Probably no other disease diagnosis causes as much horror to a previously healthy person as does the diagnosis of cancer. It sounds like a death sentence, and indeed in some patients it will be. However, there is good news for those prepared to stop and listen and to do something for themselves. The first good news is that most cancers can be cured. Even without taking into account the common less dangerous skin cancers, BCCs and SCCs, the majority of people with cancer will be cured if they are treated by an appropriate expert or by a team of experts. It is important, however, to seek help and have treatment as early as possible in the course of the disease. The longer the delay in seeking help the more advanced the cancer will become and the more difficult it will be to cure. This applies to any cancer, but the fear of knowing and facing the diagnosis and the fear of treatment often causes people to put off doing anything about their suspected problem. Despite delay in seeking treatment many patients can still be cured, although the treatment needed may be more complex. The possibility of cure does depend on the type of cancer, the site of the cancer, the general health, well-being and cooperation of the patient, and the skills and facilities of the treatment team. However it must be stressed that the earlier diagnosis is made and the most appropriate treatment is commenced, the more likelihood there is of cure.

The next good news is that we now have a much better understanding of what cancer is and how it gets started, including something of the changes in cells and their genes that may lead to cancer. Better knowledge usually leads to better solutions.

All living plants as well as all animals are composed of living cells that are often damaged or need to be replaced when they have served their function. When a new replacement cell is needed, the process of cell division begins and a new cell is formed to keep the body living and functioning normally. This process is under the control of genes in the cell nucleus. The genes are inherited from parents and bestow particular features in the offspring, such as height, skin colour, eye colour, blood group and countless other functions and distinctive features, including promotion and control of the development of new cells when they are needed. This process is normally under remarkably well-balanced control. A cancer forms when something changes in one or more of these cells: they continue to divide and divide again, producing more abnormal cells that still continue to divide and increase in number when they are not needed. The masses of unwanted dividing cells cause damage to other cells and tissues in the body.

It seems that either an abnormal gene has been inherited or something has caused one of the genes to go wrong and behave badly. There are limitless factors that can play a part in causing damage to cells and their genes. Studies will continue to try to discover why and how the ultimate change happens to make a cell become malignant. One obvious factor is that the longer we live the more often cells and the genes in them will have divided and the more likely it is that something might go wrong in the dividing process. So most cancers become more common the longer we live, in old age. Another factor is the rate of division for growth or replacement of tissues. Tissues like skin, stomach or bowel lining, or lining of the air passages in lungs, and also blood cells are constantly being shed and replenished; breast cells are constantly changing due to hormone activity over a woman's fertile period so that there is more likelihood of a mistake being made in the billions of processes of cell division (a mistake called genetic mutation). These then are the tissues most likely to undergo malignant change. Bone cancer is most likely to develop in growing young people when their bones are growing. Testicular cell activity is greatest in young adult males during the period when male sex hormones are most active, and these are the times of life most prone to these cancers. As men grow old the slow but constant changes in the prostate gland make it more likely that factors causing a change in cells might go wrong after years of exposure to the driving force of male hormones. So prostate cancer becomes increasingly common in old age.

The remarkable thing is not that something goes wrong with the delicate process of cell division, but that things don't go wrong more often. The better we look after our bodies with good living practices— including good nutrition, avoiding exposure to potentially damaging agents, regular healthy exercise and detecting and fixing anything that may be starting to go wrong—the greater is the likelihood of preventing something from seriously going awry. The body is composed of many billions of different cells, some needing to be replaced frequently, others not so often, but each time there is cell division there is a potential chance that something could go wrong.

Cancer prevention is about giving our bodies the best possible chance to get on with the normal living process and especially to avoid anything likely to upset the delicate precision of the divisions of billions of cells needed for growth, repair and healthy body activity and function. We should try to keep fit and active and not do anything to abuse or prevent this everyday process from continuing normally. We should not add known noxious chemical or physical agents like tobacco or damaging irradiation. We should provide our bodies with their most needed nutritional ingredients in our diets and avoid anything known to be potentially damaging.

We have learned a lot from these and other studies. There is much good news—more exciting news is that with present day knowledge and initiation of good health practices in everyday living, the risk of getting a cancer can be very greatly reduced. Some cancers can be largely avoided. We don't know it all yet, but we do not have to wait for further molecular and scientific discoveries to take very effective measures in reducing the risk of cancer. Much can be done with present-day knowledge. Even the single practice of not smoking will at least halve the risk of contracting several of the more prevalent and more dangerous cancers. By taking protection against excessive UV irradiation and paying attention to good dietary practices many more cancers can be avoided, or at least made less likely. By detecting and removing potentially malignant lesions before any cancer has developed in them, yet another group of cancers can be avoided. In many areas of cancer prevention people can develop their own good lifestyle practices and hopefully set examples for their children to follow. In some areas such as in cancer screening programmes to detect early and curable lesions, three way cooperation between people at risk, state health authorities and medical practitioners is needed.

With further studies and increasing knowledge more will be learnt about avoiding cancer, but much is already known. It is now up to us, each one of us, to make simple adjustments to our lifestyles. More importantly it is up to each of us to set good examples to our children and young people so that good cancer prevention practices will be natural to them and to subsequent generations.

It cannot be overemphasized that:

The best thing we can do about cancer is to do everything we can not to get one.

Addendum

Much of the improved knowledge of cancer prevention and treatment is a result of intensive and
dedicated study and research. This is expensive and
requires skilled and dedicated workers and first class
facilities, but good research must be supported as
much as possible. However there are occasions when
incidental or accidental observations have indicated
valuable potential ways of improvement, and there
are some notable examples of this in cancer research.

An astute follow-up of an incidental observation
has led to widespread use of aspirin. Precursors of
aspirin were accidentally discovered in the bark of a
tree by German scientists about 200 years ago.
Aspirin was later brought to common clinical practice by the Bayer company as a simple but effective
pain relieving agent. After years of use it was noticed
that aspirin had side effects, one of which was
increased risk of bleeding. Studies then showed that
aspirin reduced blood clotting. This side effect of

aspirin was found to be valuable in treating a number of heart and blood vessel health problems. To achieve anti-clotting benefits only a very small daily dose of aspirin is needed, and such small doses are now widely used for the anti-clotting qualities. With this widespread use it was incidentally observed only a few years ago that people taking a small daily dose of aspirin also have a lower risk of developing a bowel cancer. This has now been put to clinical use as a preventive measure for bowel cancer, one of the most common cancers in the Western world.

Some years ago an accidental injection of an anti-cancer drug into an artery rather than into a vein resulted in an increased local drug reaction. This happened in an American clinic and the clinic chief was astute enough to appreciate that the intense localized reaction seen after this clinical accident could be put to clinical advantage. In treating some patients with locally advanced or aggressive cancers, infusion of anti-cancer drugs directly into an artery supplying the cancer with blood led to a greater reaction and destruction of the cancers. Thus he developed a technique of more effective use of some anti-cancer drugs to make a locally advanced cancer smaller when given pre-operatively directly into its artery of blood supply. We in the Sydney University Surgical Oncology Clinics and others have capitalized on this to make treatment of some cancers considerably more effective. In many cases, large and aggressive cancers can be reduced to smaller and less aggressive tumours by chemotherapy, given as the first part of an integrated plan of treatment. In some instances the cancers can be so reduced in size and aggressive qualities that they are made more curable by surgery and/or the radiotherapy that then follows. If the chemotherapy can be given directly into the artery that supplies blood to the cancer, with many drugs, their increased local concentration can make them more effective with a greater likelihood of cure by following surgery or radiotherapy.

Breast cancer and prostate cancer are known to be associated with excessive or prolonged activity of female or male hormones. Asian women and Asian men have a lower incidence of breast and prostate cancers than women and men in Western countries. Recent studies have shown that plant hormones, called phytoestrogens, could counter the effect of excessive animal hormones. This was confirmed from observations that sheep and cattle grazing on pastures of clover appeared to thrive well physically, but showed hormonal changes associated with large amounts of plant hormones (phytoestrogens). It was also appreciated that the traditional diets of Asian men and women have a high content of plant hormones that counter the effects of excessive human hormones. All plants have phytoestrogens, but legumes of the pea and bean families have high levels. Legumes like soy and beans with high phytoestrogen content are an essential part of Asian diets. In Western countries diets contain much less plant food and greater amounts of meat, animal fat and dairy products with very little phytoestrogen.

Clover, like soy, is a legume and all legumes contain plentiful phytoestrogens. The red clover has about 10 times the equivalent amount present in soy and also has a larger range of active phytoestrogen components called isoflavones, and other related compounds.

Australian teams developed a technique for extracting phytoestrogens from red clover, and two or three companies now market the products in tablet form. One product has an equivalent amount of phytoestrogens in one tablet to that present in a regular healthy Asian daily diet. In these doses no unwanted side-effects of phytoestrogens have been found, but other studies are now showing other potential desirable properties of these agents. Of greatest interest to this writer is their possible potential role in cancer prevention, particularly breast cancer and prostate cancer. However the important phytoestrogen isoflavones of red clover (Genistein, Daidsein, Biochanin A, and Formonetin) now appear to have a range of other medicinal qualities including possibly relieving symptoms of pre-menstrual tension and menopausal hot flushes. Other potential benefits appear to be an ability to reduce the risk of osteoporosis, and to help normalize blood pressure and reduce other vascular problems. These aspects are all under investigation, but no definite conclusions have yet been formed.

Thus while most progress in research, including cancer research, is made by scientists working in expensively equipped laboratories, in many cases astute observations made by thoughtful people in everyday situations can provide clues to a new or different approach that merits further study. It is important to listen to what people have to say about their observations, and to think about old or traditional treatments used in different cultures. They are not all full of magic but some will still have something important to offer.

Clinical trials

Before clinical progress can be made, all theories and observations need confirmatory evidence of properly conducted clinical trials. These are studies in the care of patients who agree to take part in comparing two methods of investigation or treatment. In most cases one group is treated by the best known method. The other group is treated by a method that has not yet been proven although strong evidence suggests that it may have an advantage. Results of the two methods of treatment are compared. Such studies should always be conducted under well supervised conditions by experts in the field, most often in a teaching hospital or clinic. Patients who agree to take part will know that they will be helping to make important progress in the field, and that no matter which arm of treatment they are given they will receive the highest standards of care. Such trials are conducted all over the world and they have made, and continue to make, important contributions in prevention and treatment of many health problems, including cancer. These types of strictly controlled research studies are used to confirm or put to rest old beliefs or new theories. Thus progress is made. Results are not just an accidental or one off experience but are almost certainly reproducible under similar circumstances. This is the basis of a recently adopted phrase to describe such information—'evidence based medicine'.

Unfortunately, reliable research information takes time, patience, cooperation between study groups and the considerable cooperation of people under study. It is also expensive. Despite this, real and reliable progress is being made, in many aspects of medicine, including cancer prevention and the care of people with cancer. There is still a long way to go, but genuine improvements in recent years make it all very much worthwhile.

As I wrote at the beginning of this book, all workers in cancer research have the objective of making themselves redundant by eliminating this scourge of disease from all communities. It has always been a privilege to work in this field, and to be able to write this book, which spreads good news of progress.

Glossary

Acute Sudden; having a sudden, severe and short course.

Adenoma A benign (not malignant) tumour in which the cells are derived from glands or from glandular epithelium such as the lining of the stomach or bowel.

Anorexia Lack or loss of appetite for food.

Aspiration Act of sucking up, sucking in or sucking out, usually with a needle and syringe.

Atrophy Wasting away, losing special qualities. (Verb or noun.)

Axilla Armpit.

Bacteria Germs.

Barrett's oesophagus An inflammed lower oesophagus due to regurgitation of food and gastric juices from the stomach into the oesophagus. It may develop into a Barrett's ulcer or possibly a cancer.

Barrett's ulcer An ulcer that sometimes occurs in the lower oesophagus due to regurgitation of food and gastric juices from the stomach into the lower oesophagus. The ulcer was first described by an Australian surgeon, Dr Barrett, working in London.

Basal Basic, the lowest or foundation part of a structure. The basal layer of skin cells consist of the deep cells from which the upper or more superficial surface cells grow.

Basal cell carcinoma (BCC) Slowly growing skin cancer that has grown from the deep (basal) layer of skin cells.

Benign Not malignant; favourable for recovery and unlikely to be dangerous.

Biopsy The removal of a small sample of a tissue for microscopic examination.

Buccal mucosa The lining of the cheek in the mouth.

Cancer A malignant growth of cells. A continuous, purposeless, unwanted, uncontrolled and destructive growth of cells.

Capsule The fibrous or membranous sac-like covering that encloses a tissue or organ.

Carcinogen A substance that causes cancer.

CAT See CT.

Cervix uteri The neck of the uterus; the entrance of the womb.

Chemotherapy Treatment with chemical agents or drugs.

Chronic   Persisting for a long time, having a long or protracted course.

Chronic atrophic gastritis   Gradual and persistent degeneration of the lining of the stomach.

Congenital   Present from the time of birth.

Crohn's disease   Granular colitis, an inflammation affecting the large bowel or a similar inflammatory condition that may affect the small intestine. It was first described by Dr Kennedy Dalziel in Scotland in 1913 and later extensively studied and reported by Dr Crohn in the USA.

CT scan, CAT scan or Computerized Axial Tomography   A method of visualizing body tissues by using special computerized radiographic techniques. These give X-ray images of sections of body tissues.

Cytotoxic   Having a toxic or harmful affect upon cells.

DNA   Deoxyribonucleic acid—the material from which the body building genes and chromosomes are made.

Dysplastic   An abnormal development. Dysplastic moles are moles with unusual appearance and often other unusual features.

Endoscope   An instrument used for looking at the interior of hollow organs (such as the stomach or bowel), or the interior of body cavities (such as the abdominal cavity or chest cavity).

Epidemiology   The branch of medicine dealing with the distribution of disease and causes and spread of diseases.

Epithelium A surface lining of cells covering skin or the internal lining of hollow body organs such as the mouth, stomach, bowel, uterus, vagina or bladder or the lining of a duct like a breast duct.

Epidemiological To do with epidemiology.

Esophagus See oesophagus.

Faeces Bowel motion, stool.

Familial polyposis coli An inherited condition in which about half of the members of a family will develop polyps (small tumours) in the wall of the large bowel. Eventually one or more of these will become malignant.

Fascia Superficial fascia: the fatty layer under the skin; deep fascia: the fibrous or membranous layer of tissue that covers muscles, nerves and blood vessels, or separates muscles or other tissues into different compartments.

Fibroma A benign tumour composed of fibrous tissues and fibrous tissue-forming cells.

Floor of mouth The lower part of the mouth under the tongue.

Gastroscope An instrument used for visual examination of the interior of the stomach. See endoscope.

Genetic Inherited. A feature inherited through a gene taken from a parent.

Gland A tissue or organ that manufactures and secretes chemical substances necessary for maintenance of normal health and body function.

Glucan A complex carbohydrate (type of sugar) that constitutes much of the fibre in common vegetable and grain foodstuffs. It has also been found to have immune stimulatory properties.

Goitre   Enlargement of the thyroid gland causing a swelling in the lower front part of the neck.

Granular colitis   A chronic inflammatory condition of the large bowel of no known cause, first reported by Dr Dalziel in Scotland but extensively studied and described by Dr Crohn in America. (See Crohn's Disease.)

HRT (hormone replacement therapy)   Treatment with a low dose of hormones given to reduce menopausal and postmenopausal symptoms and other associated problems such as loss of calcium from bones.

Hyperkeratosis   A thickening of the flat protective surface layer of epithelium of skin or lip. The condition is usually characterized by the formation of crusts or flakes that drop off and then recur. There is a tendency for malignant changes to appear gradually and thus a cancer may develop.

Induration   The hardening or thickening of a tissue or a part of the body due to inflammation or infiltration with cancer.

Infiltrating or invasive   When used in reference to cancer, these terms describe cancers with cells that gradually permeate or creep into surrounding tissues.

In situ   When used in reference to cancer this describes a cancer that is composed of cancer cells that have remained localized and not spread into adjacent or surrounding tissues.

Isoflavones   A class of plant hormones (phytoestrogens) that are present in many plants but especially plentiful in legume plants like soya beans. The greatest known source is in the red clover plant. The red clover is a legume that contains all the phytoestrogens known to be active in human physiology.

Legume A class of plant that includes members of the bean and pea families. All plants of this type contain relatively large amounts of the isoflavonoid phytoestrogens.

Lesion An abnormal area of tissue or a localized area of tissue damage.

Leucocyte White cell. The 'white' or colourless type of cell that circulates in the blood, has amoeboid movement, and is chiefly concerned with defending the body against invasion by foreign organisms or bacteria or foreign materials.

Leukoplakia White patch. A disease distinguished by the presence of white thickened patches in the mucous membranes, commonly in the mouth. There may be a tendency for malignant characteristics to appear gradually and thus for a cancer to develop.

Lipoma A benign tumour or lump composed of fat cells.

Liver The largest solid organ in the body. It lies in the upper abdomen predominantly on the right side and under cover of the lower right ribs.

Lymphocyte One of the types of white cells that circulate in the blood and take part in immune reactions and the body's defence reactions. It is a mononuclear (single nucleus) non-granular leucocyte and is produced by lymph nodes and other lymphoid tissue as well as by bone marrow.

Lymphoid   Resembling or pertaining to the tissue of the lymphatic system. Tissue that contains large numbers of round cells and produces lymphocytes and is part of the immune system.

Lymphoma   A neoplastic disease or cancer of lymphoid tissue.

Lymph nodes   Small masses of lymphatic tissue 1–25 mm diameter and normally bean-shaped. They are scattered along the course of lymph vessels and often grouped in clusters. They form an important part of the body's defence system. They function as factories for the development of lymphocytes and filter bacteria and foreign debris from tissue fluid. They are not glands but are sometimes called lymph glands.

Lymph vessels or lymphatics   The small vessels that drain tissue fluid into lymph nodes and interconnect groups of lymph nodes. Eventually the larger lymph vessels drain this fluid into the blood stream.

Mammogram   Special X-rays of the breast in which very small doses of X-rays are used to show tissues of different densities in the breasts.

Malaise   A general feeling of lassitude and ill-health; feeling unwell.

Malignant   Having progressive and threatening qualities.

Melanoma   A malignant tumour of pigment-producing cells most commonly arising in the skin, sometimes in the eye and occasionally elsewhere.

Metastasis   Metastatic cancer—a secondary growth or seeding of malignant cells that has spread from a primary cancer elsewhere.

MRI (magnetic resonance imaging)   A special test based on magnetic laws of physics. The test allows very detailed X-ray-like pictures to be taken of cross sections of the body, head or limbs. The resulting pictures are rather like those of CT scans.

Mucus   A protective slimy material secreted by certain glands and certain cells lining body cavities and hollow organs.

Mucus membrane   The lining of most hollow organs and some body cavities such as the mouth, stomach and bowel, all of which contain mucous glands and secrete mucus onto the surface.

Naevus (or nevus)   A localized collection of pigment-forming skin cells forming a localized and circumscribed malformation, usually pigmented brown in colour, for example a mole or a birthmark.

Neoplasm (new growth)   An abnormal growth of body cells. A neoplasm may be benign (innocent and usually harmless) with limited growth, or malignant (cancer) with continuous, unwanted, unlimited, uncontrolled and destructive growth.

Neuroma   A benign tumour composed of nerve cells.

Oesophagus (or esophagus)   The part of the digestive tract for passage of food from the mouth and pharynx above to the stomach below. It is a muscular tube with a lining of flat epithelial cells like skin surface cells and extends from the neck, through the chest and into the abdomen to join the stomach.

Oncology   The study of tumours or of patients suffering from tumours.

Pap smear test   A test for cancer cells or pre-cancer cells in the cervix of the uterus. Named after the Greek doctor Papanicolaou who first described this cancer detection test.

Pancreas   A pale fleshy gland that lies across the back of the abdominal cavity, mostly behind the stomach. It is responsible for secreting digestive juices into the digestive tract and for the secretion of insulin into the blood stream.

Papilloma   A benign wart-like or fern-like tumour derived from epithelial cells like skin or duct surface cells and projecting from an epithelial surface with a central core of small blood vessels.

PET scan (positron emission tomography)   A special technique of giving 'pictures' of body tissues based on different biochemical activity of sugars in the tissues. Cancer cells use more sugar (glucose) than normal cells and therefore show up differently in PET scans.

Physiology   The study of normal function of the body.

Physiological   Having to do with normal body chemistry and function.

Phytoestrogens   Naturally occurring oestrogen-like hormones present in all plants but in relatively large quantities in certain leguminous plants such as soy beans. Thought to be at least partly responsible for the lower incidence of some cancers (especially of breast and prostate) in people such as Asians who have a high intake of legumes in their diets.

Pleura   The lining or membrane surrounding the lungs and the cavity in which the lungs move during breathing.

Polyp   A tumour projecting on a stalk from the mucous membrane lining the cavity of a hollow organ.

PMS (postmenopausal syndrome)   Symptoms of hot flushes, depression, vaginal dryness, bone wasting (osteoporosis) etc. associated with menopausal changes.

Pre-invasive   In reference to cancer this describes a cancer with cells that appear to be malignant but have not yet begun to infiltrate or spread into surrounding tissues. An *in situ* cancer or a latent cancer.

Prostate   A small gland in males that stimulates spermatozoa to make them fertile in their passage from the testes to the penis. It is about the size and shape of a walnut and situated deep in the pelvis at the base of the bladder.

PSA (prostate specific antigen)   The PSA test is a blood test to determine the amount of this special enzyme in the blood. This enzyme is produced by prostate gland cells and when the number of these cells is increased there is usually a raised level in the blood. High PSA levels can be an indication of the presence of prostate cancer although other non-malignant conditions, especially prostate hyperplasia, can also cause the PSA to be raised.

Radical   Extreme or very extensive. A radical mastectomy is removal of the whole breast together with other nearby tissues.

Red clover A type of clover plant that contains the highest known concentration of the isoflavonoid phytoestrogens.

Sarcoma A cancer of connective tissues such as muscle, fat, fascia or bone.

Screening test A relatively simple, safe and easily performed test that can be carried out on large numbers of people to determine whether they are likely to have a cancer or other serious disease.

Sigmoidoscope A long, thin, hollow instrument used for passing through the anus with a light to allow visual examination of the inside of the lower bowel.

Soy An extract of the soya bean.

Soya bean A commonly eaten bean, rich in protein and carbohydrate, that contains relatively large quantities of the isoflavonoid phytoestrogens. Soya beans are easily grown and cheaply produced legumes. They are thus a cheap but nourishing food and an important part of traditional diets in many countries, especially in Asia.

Squamous Flat, like a scale or pavement. Squamous cells are flat scale-like cells that cover the skin, the mouth, throat, oesophagus, vagina and some other cavities.

Therapy Treatment.

Tissue A layer or group of cells of particular specialized types that together make a special part or perform a special function.

Toxic   Poisonous.

Trauma   Injury.

Traumatized   Injured.

Tumour   A swelling. Commonly used to describe a swelling caused by a growth of cells—a new growth (neoplasm) may be benign or may be a cancer.

Ulcerative colitis   An inflammatory condition of the large bowel with small ulcers in the bowel lining and causing episodes of diarrhoea, sometimes with blood loss.

Uterus   The womb. The organ in the female pelvis in which a baby (or fetus) develops.

Varicose ulcer   An ulcer in the skin, usually on the lower leg, caused by poor circulation in the tissues due to long standing varicose veins.

Index

Index